FamilyPro Guide to
Pregnancy Nutrition and Diet

The Ultimate Handbook to Healthy Eating While Expecting

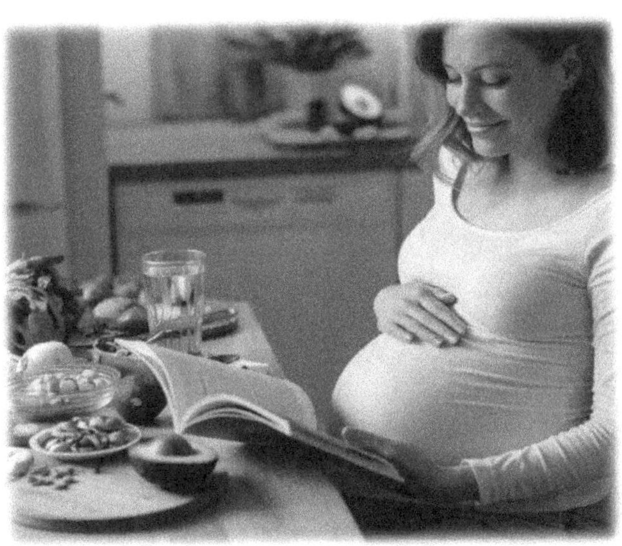

Raquel Allen

Table of Contents

Introduction

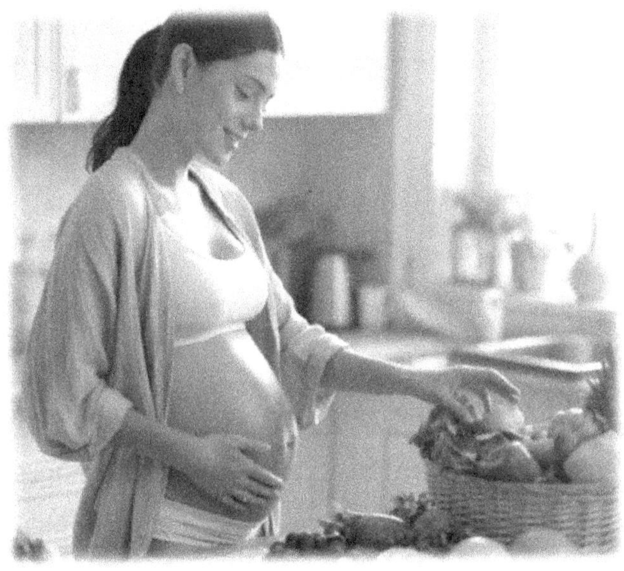

Pregnancy is one of life's most profound journeys, a time brimming with anticipation, hope, and transformation. It's a season when excitement often mingles with anxiety, and joy walks hand in hand with the unknown. From the moment you discover you're expecting, your world changes forever. Suddenly, every decision, every choice—especially when it comes to food and nourishment—takes on a new depth of importance. You find yourself wondering if you're doing everything right, if you're giving your growing baby the best possible start, and if you have what it takes to thrive through this beautiful, challenging time.

The physical changes that come with pregnancy are incredible and, at times, overwhelming. Your body, the very core of who you are, adapts and stretches in ways you never imagined possible. You may feel an entirely new spectrum of emotions, from boundless energy to overwhelming fatigue, and everything in between. There are days of radiant energy and strength, where you feel deeply connected to your baby and inspired by the miracle of life within. And there are days when you feel exhausted, battling morning sickness or aches, just hoping for relief. Each of these feelings is normal; each is part of this powerful experience.

If there's one area that brings both a sense of control and confusion, it's nutrition. Eating becomes more than just feeding yourself—it's about nourishing the tiny being who depends on you for every vitamin, mineral, and nutrient they need to grow. Yet, with every well-meaning suggestion and flood of online advice, it can feel difficult to discern what truly matters. Questions arise: What should I eat to feel better? What's safe? How can I manage cravings, or balance my growing appetite with good choices? It's easy to feel lost in this new world of nutritional needs and dietary "rules."

This is where knowledge becomes your ally, and this book is here to provide that knowledge in a way that empowers you, reassures you, and simplifies the complex world of pregnancy nutrition. You don't need to have all the answers; you just need a reliable guide—a trusted companion that helps you make informed decisions without adding unnecessary stress. This book aims to be that guide, walking with you every step of the way, giving you the insights you need to make choices that feel right for you and your baby.

Pregnancy isn't a one-size-fits-all experience, and your nutritional needs are as unique as your journey. We know that each trimester brings its own set of challenges and joys, and each stage of your pregnancy will shape the way you eat, the foods you crave, and even the foods you can tolerate. Early on, you might be facing morning sickness or unusual cravings, and later, you might find yourself eating a little more to meet your growing energy needs. As your pregnancy progresses, your baby's needs change too. Their tiny bones need calcium, their muscles need protein, and their developing brain relies on nutrients like Omega-3 fatty acids. Through each chapter of this book, you'll find guidance tailored to these unique needs, helping you feel confident in the choices you make at every step.

This book isn't just about what foods to eat or avoid; it's also about the "why" behind these recommendations. With a clear understanding of the reasons behind each choice, you can embrace each meal as an opportunity to care for both yourself and your baby. There's a particular power in knowing that your breakfast, lunch, and dinner are working for you, enhancing your health, supporting your baby's growth, and even uplifting your mood. You'll learn to select foods that support your energy and well-being, helping you feel grounded on days when things feel chaotic or overwhelming.

And let's not forget about joy. Food, after all, is meant to be enjoyed. While you're learning what's best for your body and baby, you'll also discover ways to savor your meals, indulge your cravings, and build a relationship with food that feels satisfying and nourishing. From hearty breakfasts that keep nausea at bay, to comforting dinners that help you unwind, to snacks that lift your spirits during long afternoons—this book is filled with practical tips and enjoyable recipes. These pages will remind you that eating during pregnancy is as much about savoring the moment as it is about the nutrients you're taking in.

Above all, know that every choice you make in caring for yourself and your baby is a testament to your strength and love. The fact that you're here, reading these words, shows that you're ready to take on this responsibility with grace and commitment. Pregnancy can often bring moments of self-doubt, and it's normal to feel unsure about whether you're doing enough or doing things "right." Trust that you are. Trust that your body is resilient, adaptable, and capable of guiding you through the months to come. And remember that you're not alone; countless women have walked this path, and many others are walking it with you now.

As you move forward, know that this book is here for the highs, the lows, and everything in between. It's here to encourage you, to empower you, and to give you practical answers when you feel uncertain. As you work through each chapter, you'll build a strong foundation of knowledge. You'll gain tools to nurture your body, even as it changes in ways you may not expect. You'll find answers to common concerns and discover ways to handle the inevitable challenges that come with pregnancy.

More than just a guide, think of this book as a source of comfort and strength. Let its pages reassure you on the harder days and inspire you on the good days. Embrace the knowledge within as a steadying force, reminding you that you're prepared, you're informed, and you're giving your baby the gift of mindful care. In these pages, you'll find the information you need to navigate each trimester, overcome any hurdles, and celebrate every victory.

So take a deep breath, let go of any lingering fears, and give yourself permission to enjoy this time. Pregnancy is full of surprises, both challenging and wonderful, but with each day, you're getting closer to meeting your baby. You're creating a safe, loving environment for them from the very start, one healthy meal at a time. Allow yourself to lean on the guidance this book offers, and trust that you're doing an amazing job.

You've already taken the first step by seeking out this knowledge. With every page you turn, may you feel more assured, more hopeful, and more empowered. Here's to a healthy, joyful pregnancy, and to the incredible bond you're building with your baby. Keep reading, keep learning, and know that you are more than enough. This is just the beginning of an incredible journey, one that you are more than capable of navigating with strength, wisdom, and love.

Chapter 1: The Foundations of Pregnancy Nutrition

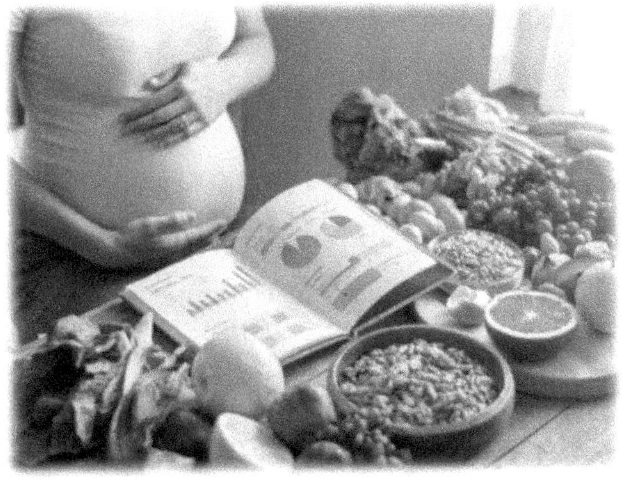

Pregnancy nutrition refers to the careful selection of foods and nutrients that support the health of both mother and baby. Proper nutrition during this time is essential, as it ensures optimal fetal development, strengthens the mother's immune system, and prepares the body for the challenges of childbirth and recovery.

The Role of Nutrition During Pregnancy

When you're pregnant, everything you eat and drink plays a direct role in the development of your baby and your own health. The way your body works during pregnancy is complex, and it's important to fuel it properly. Nutrition during pregnancy isn't just about eating more food; it's about eating the right foods in the right amounts. What you consume affects not only your body's ability to support your growing baby but also your energy levels, immune system, and overall well-being.

Your baby's growth and development rely heavily on the nutrients you provide. From the earliest stages of pregnancy, when your baby is just a tiny cluster of cells, they are using the nutrients you eat to form vital organs, tissues, and structures. A healthy diet will help ensure that your baby develops normally and that you're prepared for the physical demands of pregnancy.

Supporting Your Baby's Growth

Your baby's first and most critical developments happen during the early weeks of pregnancy. During this time, the foundation for major organs, including the heart, brain, and spinal cord, is being laid. Without the proper nutrients, these structures can develop abnormally. For example, folic acid, a B-vitamin, plays a key role in preventing neural tube defects, which affect the brain and spinal cord. That's why it's recommended to start taking a prenatal vitamin with folic acid before even trying to conceive, and continue throughout pregnancy.

As your pregnancy progresses, your baby continues to grow, gaining weight and developing important body systems. The nutrients you eat now are crucial for this continued growth. Proteins are essential for building muscle, skin, and internal organs. Calcium is vital for strong bones and teeth, and iron helps with the production of hemoglobin, which carries oxygen to your baby's tissues. A deficiency in these nutrients could lead to complications like low birth weight or preterm birth, as well as affecting your own health.

Maintaining Your Health During Pregnancy

The role of nutrition during pregnancy isn't just about your baby—it's equally important for you. Pregnancy puts a lot of strain on your body. Your body is working overtime to support your growing baby, which means it requires more of certain nutrients than before. This includes increased amounts of iron (to prevent anemia), calcium (to support bone health), and protein (for overall tissue growth). Proper nutrition also helps keep you energized, helps your immune system stay strong, and aids in managing common pregnancy discomforts like nausea and constipation.

Your diet can also cause certain pregnancy-related conditions. For example, gestational diabetes, which is a type of diabetes that develops during pregnancy, can often be managed or even prevented with proper diet and regular physical activity. Similarly, preeclampsia, a condition that causes high blood pressure, can sometimes be controlled when you reduce sodium intake and consume a well-balanced diet.

The Importance of a Balanced Diet

Eating a balanced diet means choosing foods from all the food groups: fruits, vegetables, whole grains, proteins, and dairy. Each of these food groups provides essential nutrients your body needs to keep both you and your baby healthy. A diet that's too high in processed foods, sugars, or fats can lead to excess weight gain or nutritional deficiencies. So, focus on variety and nutrient-dense foods.

For instance, fruits and vegetables are rich in vitamins and antioxidants, which help protect both you and your baby from inflammation and infections. Whole grains provide fiber and B-vitamins, which are important for digestion and energy. Lean proteins like chicken, beans, and fish are crucial for tissue growth and development. Dairy products are key sources of calcium, which supports your baby's bone development and your own bone health.

Hydration is Key

Water is often overlooked in pregnancy nutrition, but it's one of the most important things you can consume. Hydration is essential for supporting the increased blood volume in your body, as well as maintaining amniotic fluid levels. Dehydration can lead to fatigue, headaches, and even premature labor. Make sure to drink plenty of water throughout the day—at least 8-10 cups. Try to avoid sugary drinks or caffeine, as they can dehydrate you.

Nutrition and Emotional Well-Being

Good nutrition also plays a role in your emotional health during pregnancy. Hormonal changes can make you feel more stressed or anxious at times, and the foods you eat can help stabilize your mood. Omega-3 fatty acids, found in fish like salmon, are known to support brain health and can even help reduce feelings of anxiety. Magnesium, found in leafy greens, nuts, and seeds, can promote relaxation and better sleep. Balanced blood sugar levels from whole, unprocessed foods also help keep your energy levels stable, which can prevent mood swings.

Practical Tips for Getting It Right

Nutrition during pregnancy doesn't have to be complicated. Small, practical changes to your diet can make a huge difference for both you and your baby.

- Plan meals ahead to ensure you're getting a variety of nutrients throughout the day.
- Eat smaller, more frequent meals to keep your blood sugar stable and avoid nausea.
- Take a prenatal vitamin to fill any gaps in your nutrition.

- Choose healthy snacks like nuts, yogurt, or fruit instead of sugary treats.
- Drink plenty of water to stay hydrated and avoid dehydration.

Conclusion

The role of nutrition during pregnancy is vital for your health and your baby's development. Choose a variety of nutrient-rich foods and staying hydrated to ensure that your pregnancy is as healthy as possible. Good nutrition will not only support your baby's growth but also help you manage the physical and emotional demands of pregnancy.

Strategic Suggestions

Focus on eating nutrient-dense, whole foods. You can stay hydrated, aiming for 8-10 cups of water daily. Incorporating omega-3-rich foods like salmon into your diet would also help. Consider opting for small, frequent meals to help manage nausea and maintain energy. Remember to take your prenatal vitamin based on your healthcare provider's recommendation.

Taking these steps will help you feel your best during pregnancy and give your baby the nutrients they need to thrive.

Key Nutrients for a Healthy Pregnancy

When you're pregnant, your body's nutritional needs change to support the rapid growth and development of your baby. Providing your body with the right balance of vitamins, minerals, and other nutrients is essential. These nutrients not only help your baby grow but also ensure that you stay healthy and energized throughout your pregnancy. Let's explore the key nutrients you need, why they matter, and how you can get them.

Folic Acid: The Building Block for Your Baby's Development

One of the first nutrients to focus on when you're planning to get pregnant is folic acid, a B-vitamin that is critical for your baby's early development. Folic acid helps prevent neural tube defects, which are serious birth defects that affect the brain and spinal cord. This is especially important in the first few weeks of pregnancy, often before you even know you're pregnant. For this reason, doctors recommend that you start taking a prenatal vitamin with folic acid even before conception, and continue through the first trimester.

To ensure you're getting enough folic acid, aim for at least 400-800 micrograms daily. You can get folic acid from fortified cereals, leafy greens like spinach and kale, legumes, and citrus fruits. It's a simple nutrient to get, but it's vital for early brain and spinal cord development.

Iron: Vital for Oxygen and Blood Production

During pregnancy, your body's blood volume increases to supply oxygen and nutrients to your growing baby. As a result, you need more iron to help produce extra red blood cells. Iron is crucial for the production of hemoglobin, the protein in red blood cells that carries oxygen from your lungs to the rest of your body and to your baby.

Iron deficiency can lead to anemia, which can cause fatigue, weakness, and a higher risk of complications during childbirth. Pregnant women need around 27 milligrams of iron per day—almost double the amount recommended for women who aren't pregnant.

Good sources of iron include lean meats like beef and chicken, as well as plant-based sources like lentils, beans, tofu, and fortified cereals. Iron is better absorbed when consumed with vitamin C, so try pairing iron-rich foods with foods like oranges, strawberries, or bell peppers.

Calcium: Building Strong Bones and Teeth

Calcium is essential for the development of your baby's bones and teeth, and it's just as important for your own bone health, especially since your body is working harder to support your growing baby. If you don't consume enough calcium during pregnancy, your body will take it from your bones to meet your baby's needs, which can lead to bone density loss over time.

Pregnant women need about 1,000 milligrams of calcium per day, which increases to 1,300 milligrams if you're under 19. Dairy products like milk, yogurt, and cheese are rich sources of calcium, but if you're lactose intolerant or prefer plant-based options, you can also get calcium from fortified plant milks (like almond, soy, or oat), leafy greens, tofu, and almonds.

Protein: Supporting Growth and Repair

Protein is the building block of your baby's cells, tissues, muscles, and organs. It's essential for both your baby's growth and your body's increased energy needs. Protein also helps with the repair of tissues and helps to form enzymes and hormones needed for your body to function properly during pregnancy.

Pregnant women need about 71 grams of protein per day. Great sources of protein include lean meats like chicken and turkey, fish, eggs, beans, lentils, nuts, seeds, and dairy. If you're a vegetarian or vegan, make sure to combine different plant-based proteins like beans, quinoa, and soy to get the full range of essential amino acids.

Vitamin D: Supporting Bone Health and Immune Function

Vitamin D is important for both you and your baby because it helps your body absorb calcium. It also plays a role in regulating your immune system and maintaining a healthy pregnancy. A deficiency in vitamin D during pregnancy has been linked to complications such as preeclampsia, gestational diabetes, and low birth weight.

You can get vitamin D through sunlight exposure, but it's also found in certain foods. Fatty fish like salmon and mackerel, fortified dairy products, and egg yolks are good sources. If you're not getting enough vitamin D from your diet or sunlight, your doctor may recommend a supplement.

Omega-3 Fatty Acids: Supporting Brain and Eye Development

Omega-3 fatty acids, particularly DHA (docosahexaenoic acid), are crucial for the development of your baby's brain, eyes, and nervous system. DHA also supports your baby's cognitive development and can even have benefits for your own mental health, potentially lowering the risk of postpartum depression.

Pregnant women are advised to get at least 200 milligrams of DHA per day. You can find omega-3 fatty acids in fatty fish like salmon, sardines, and trout, as well as in flaxseeds, walnuts, and chia seeds. If you're not consuming enough of these foods, your doctor may recommend a fish oil or algae-based DHA supplement.

Iodine: Supporting Thyroid Function

Iodine is important for the proper functioning of your thyroid, which helps regulate your metabolism and supports the development of your baby's brain and nervous system. A deficiency in iodine can lead to developmental delays and other complications, so it's crucial to make sure you're getting enough.

Pregnant women need about 220 micrograms of iodine per day. Good sources of iodine include iodized salt, dairy products, seafood, and seaweed. If you're concerned about getting enough iodine, ask your doctor if you should be using iodized salt or taking an iodine supplement.

Hydration: Keeping Everything Moving

While hydration might not technically be a "nutrient," it's still a critical part of a healthy pregnancy. Water helps maintain the increased blood volume, supports the transport of nutrients to your baby, and helps in the production of amniotic fluid. Staying hydrated also helps prevent constipation and swelling, two common pregnancy complaints.

Aim to drink 8-10 cups of water a day. If you're exercising or it's hot outside, you'll need to drink more to stay hydrated.

Strategic Suggestions

- **Eat a variety of nutrient-rich foods:** Incorporate plenty of fruits, vegetables, whole grains, and lean proteins into your daily meals.
- **Include vitamin C** with iron-rich foods to improve absorption.
- **Take a prenatal vitamin** to fill in any gaps in your diet, especially for folic acid, iodine, and iron.
- **Consider omega-3 supplements** if you're not eating enough fatty fish or plant-based omega-3 sources.
- **Monitor calcium intake**, especially if you're avoiding dairy. Aim for plant-based calcium sources or fortified foods.

Meeting these nutritional needs during pregnancy will not only give your baby the best start but also help you stay healthy and energized. A balanced diet, rich in key nutrients, is the foundation for a healthy pregnancy and a strong, healthy baby.

The Importance of Balanced Meals for Expecting Mothers

When you're pregnant, it's crucial to eat a variety of nutrient-rich foods to keep both you and your baby healthy. A balanced diet during pregnancy ensures that your baby receives all the vitamins, minerals, and energy needed for growth, while also supporting your physical health and well-being. However, simply eating more food isn't enough. What matters most is the quality of the food you eat. Proper nutrition goes beyond the idea of "eating for two"—it's about fueling your body with the right foods at the right times.

What Does a Balanced Meal Look Like During Pregnancy?

A balanced meal during pregnancy includes foods from all the major food groups: fruits, vegetables, protein sources, whole grains, and dairy or dairy alternatives. Each of these groups provides essential nutrients that your body needs in greater amounts during pregnancy. The key is variety—by choosing a mix of foods, you ensure that you get all the vitamins and minerals required to support both you and your baby.

Here's a breakdown of the components of a balanced meal for pregnancy:

1. Protein

Protein is vital for both the growth of your baby's tissues and the maintenance of your own body's functions. During pregnancy, you need about 71 grams of protein per day. Good sources include lean meats like chicken or turkey, fish, eggs, beans, tofu, nuts, and seeds. Protein-rich foods help you feel fuller for longer and provide the necessary building blocks for muscle and organ growth in your baby.

2. Whole Grains

Whole grains like brown rice, quinoa, oats, and whole wheat pasta are important sources of carbohydrates, which provide you with energy. They also contain fiber, which helps prevent constipation—a common issue during pregnancy. Additionally, whole grains are rich in B-vitamins, which support energy metabolism and nervous system function.

3. Fruits and Vegetables

Fruits and vegetables are packed with essential vitamins, minerals, and fiber. They are key for keeping your immune system strong and supporting healthy digestion. Aim for a variety of colors on your plate, as different colored fruits and vegetables offer different nutrients. For example, leafy greens like spinach and kale provide folate, while oranges and strawberries provide vitamin C, which helps with iron absorption.

4. Dairy or Dairy Alternatives

Dairy products are a great source of calcium, which is essential for your baby's bone and tooth development. If you're lactose intolerant or avoid dairy, look for fortified alternatives like almond milk, soy milk, or oat milk. Fortified plant-based milks contain calcium, vitamin D, and other important nutrients.

5. Healthy Fats

Healthy fats, such as those found in avocados, nuts, seeds, and oily fish like salmon, are crucial for brain development in your baby. Omega-3 fatty acids, in particular, are essential for the development of your baby's brain and eyes. These healthy fats also help regulate your hormones, improve circulation, and keep your skin healthy during pregnancy.

Why a Balanced Diet Matters During Pregnancy

Eating a balanced diet during pregnancy has a direct impact on both your health and your baby's development. A well-rounded approach ensures that you get the necessary nutrients for your body's increased energy demands and supports your baby's growth.

For example, getting enough calcium helps prevent your body from taking calcium from your bones to meet your baby's needs. Similarly, sufficient iron ensures that your blood can carry enough oxygen to your baby and helps you avoid becoming anemic, which can cause fatigue and other complications.

Maintaining a balanced diet can also help you avoid excessive weight gain and prevent complications like gestational diabetes, high blood pressure, and preeclampsia. When your blood sugar and nutrient levels are stable, you'll have more energy and be better able to cope with the physical challenges of pregnancy. A healthy diet can also reduce the likelihood of developing stretch marks or other skin issues, as proper hydration and nutrients can keep your skin elastic.

Additionally, a balanced diet helps to manage common pregnancy symptoms like nausea, heartburn, and constipation. For example, eating smaller, more frequent meals can help reduce nausea, while fiber-rich foods can alleviate constipation.

Meal Timing: The Key to Consistent Energy

Along with choosing the right foods, the timing of your meals matters. Pregnancy can bring about changes in your appetite, and fluctuating blood sugar levels can leave you feeling hungry or fatigued at odd times. Eating smaller meals throughout the day—rather than a few large meals—can help you maintain energy levels and keep your blood sugar stable.

Aim for three main meals and two to three snacks each day. This way, you avoid the hunger spikes that can lead to overeating or unhealthy food choices. Healthy snacks can include things like fruit, nuts, yogurt, or whole-grain crackers with cheese. These snacks help to keep your energy up and provide important nutrients, especially if you're feeling too nauseous to eat a full meal.

Hydration: An Essential Part of a Balanced Diet

While food is important, staying hydrated is just as crucial during pregnancy. Your body's fluid needs increase as your blood volume increases and your body works to support your baby. Aim for 8-10 cups of water per day, but you may need more if you're active or the weather is hot. Drinking enough water can help you avoid dehydration, which can cause fatigue, headaches, and constipation.

Strategic Suggestions

- **Make your plate colorful:** Aim for a variety of fruits and vegetables to ensure you're getting all the necessary vitamins and minerals.

- **Include healthy fats:** Incorporate omega-3-rich foods like fatty fish, flaxseeds, and walnuts for brain and eye development.

- **Eat small, frequent meals:** This helps stabilize blood sugar levels and keeps your energy up throughout the day.

- **Hydrate regularly:** Drink plenty of water and choose hydrating foods like watermelon and cucumbers.
- **Opt for whole grains:** Choose whole grain bread, pasta, and cereals to support digestion and provide long-lasting energy.

Focusing on balanced meals and ensuring that you're eating from all the food groups will not only nourish your baby but also support your own health during pregnancy. A well-balanced diet helps to ensure a smooth, healthy pregnancy and gives you the energy and strength you need to enjoy this exciting time.

Chapter 2: Nutritional Needs in the First Trimester

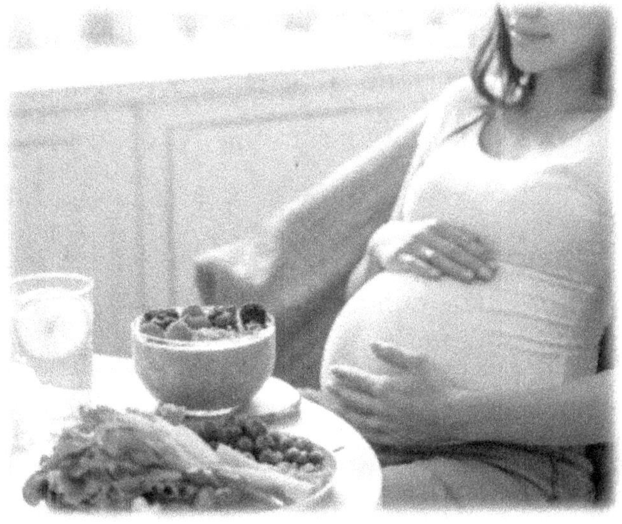

The first trimester is a crucial time for fetal development, as most major organs begin to form. Meeting the specific nutritional needs during these early weeks is vital for both the baby's growth and the mother's health, setting the foundation for a healthy pregnancy and reducing the risk of complications.

Overcoming Morning Sickness with Nutrient-Rich Foods

Morning sickness is one of the most common—and often frustrating—symptoms during the first trimester of pregnancy. It typically involves nausea and vomiting, usually in the morning but sometimes lasting all day. While the exact cause isn't entirely clear, it's thought to be related to hormonal changes and your body's adjustment to pregnancy. Eating the right types of foods at the right times can ease symptoms and ensure that both you and your baby are getting the necessary nutrients.

Understanding Morning Sickness and Its Effects on Nutrition

Morning sickness can make eating difficult, but it's important to try to nourish your body as best you can. When you're feeling nauseous, the idea of eating anything—even something that's good for you—can feel overwhelming.

However, the foods you choose can make a significant difference in how you feel.

First, it's important to acknowledge that morning sickness doesn't necessarily mean you're not eating enough. In fact, many women experience nausea and vomiting without significant weight loss. However, the key challenge is getting enough nutrients to support your baby's development and your own well-being. This is where nutrient-rich foods come into play.

Since morning sickness can lead to dehydration and nutrient imbalances, making small adjustments in what and when you eat can help manage these effects. It's all about finding foods that are easy on your stomach while still providing you with the essential nutrients your body and baby need.

Foods to Ease Nausea

When battling morning sickness, bland, easy-to-digest foods are your best friend. These foods are gentle on your stomach, help maintain your blood sugar levels, and provide a good source of the nutrients your body needs during pregnancy.

1. Ginger

One of the most popular and effective natural remedies for nausea, ginger has been shown to reduce the frequency and intensity of vomiting. You can add fresh ginger to tea, chew on ginger candies, or enjoy ginger ale (look for varieties with real ginger and low sugar).

2. Crackers and Dry Toast

Simple carbohydrates like plain crackers, dry toast, or rice cakes can absorb stomach acids and prevent nausea. These foods are mild and easy to digest, making them an ideal starting point for any meal.

3. Bananas

Rich in potassium, bananas help replenish electrolytes that might be lost due to vomiting.

They are also soft, easy on your stomach, and a source of energy that won't aggravate nausea.

4. Applesauce

The mild, sweet taste of applesauce provides a small amount of fiber and vitamin C, while being gentle on your stomach. If solid foods feel too heavy, applesauce can be a good alternative.

5. Plain Rice or Pasta

Like crackers, plain rice and pasta are simple carbohydrates that are gentle on the stomach. They provide a steady source of energy and are easy to eat without triggering nausea.

Foods to Avoid During Morning Sickness

Certain foods can worsen morning sickness or make your symptoms worse, so it's important to listen to your body and avoid them when you're feeling nauseous. Strong-smelling, spicy, or greasy foods may intensify nausea, so consider steering clear of:

1. Greasy and Fried Foods

These can be heavy and hard to digest, and may leave you feeling even more queasy.

2. Spicy Foods

Strong spices can irritate your stomach and trigger nausea.

3. Caffeinated Beverages

Coffee, sodas, and energy drinks can upset your stomach and lead to dehydration.

4. Foods with Strong Odors

Anything with a pungent smell, such as certain cheeses, meats, or garlic, can exacerbate nausea.

Hydration During Morning Sickness

Staying hydrated is essential, but when nausea strikes, drinking fluids can be difficult. Dehydration is a serious concern during this time, especially if vomiting is frequent. Sipping small amounts of water throughout the day can help, and it's a good idea to keep a bottle of water nearby to sip whenever you feel you can.

In addition to plain water, you can try:

1. Electrolyte Drinks

Low-sugar sports drinks or coconut water can help replenish lost fluids and electrolytes.

2. Herbal Teas

Peppermint and ginger teas are gentle on your stomach and can help ease nausea.

3. Ice Chips or Popsicles

These can be a refreshing way to hydrate if plain water feels unappealing.

Small, Frequent Meals

Another strategy to manage morning sickness is eating small, frequent meals throughout the day. Instead of forcing yourself to eat three large meals, try eating five or six smaller meals. This will help keep your blood sugar levels steady and prevent nausea from becoming overwhelming.

Start with easy-to-digest foods in the morning, like crackers or toast, before moving on to more substantial meals later in the day. Having a snack every 2-3 hours can also help prevent an empty stomach, which might worsen nausea.

When to Seek Help

While morning sickness is common, it can sometimes develop into a more serious condition called hyperemesis gravidarum, which causssses severe vomiting and dehydration. If you find it difficult to keep any food or liquid down, or if you experience weight loss, dizziness, or fainting, it's important to seek medical attention.

Your doctor may recommend medication or additional treatment to help control the symptoms.

Strategic Suggestions

- **Opt for bland, easy-to-digest foods** like crackers, dry toast, and rice to calm nausea.

- **Use ginger in different forms**, such as ginger tea or ginger candies, to reduce vomiting.

- **Hydrate frequently in small amounts**, using water, herbal teas, or electrolyte drinks.

- **Eat smaller, more frequent meals** to avoid an empty stomach and keep your blood sugar stable.

- **Avoid foods** with strong odors or those that are greasy, spicy, or fried.

Managing morning sickness can be challenging, but with some adjustments to your diet and meal timing, you can make this uncomfortable phase a little easier to handle. Remember, every pregnancy is different, so it's important to pay attention to how your body responds and adjust accordingly. With the right nutrient-rich foods, you can find relief and

make sure you're still nourishing both yourself
and your baby.

The Essential Role of Folic Acid and Iron

Folic acid and iron are two of the most crucial nutrients you need during the first trimester of pregnancy. Both play significant roles in supporting your health and the healthy development of your baby. Understanding their importance and ensuring you get enough of these nutrients can help you navigate this critical phase of pregnancy with confidence.

Folic Acid: The Key to Healthy Development

Folic acid, a B-vitamin, is essential for the early development of your baby, particularly during the first trimester. It plays a crucial role in the formation of the neural tube, which develops into the brain and spinal cord. Adequate folic acid intake is vital in preventing neural tube defects (NTDs) such as spina bifida and anencephaly. These defects can occur very early in pregnancy, often before you even know you're expecting.

Health professionals recommend that women who are trying to conceive or are in their first trimester consume at least 400 to 800 micrograms of folic acid daily. This can be achieved through a combination of diet and supplementation.

Sources of Folic Acid

In addition to taking prenatal vitamins, you can increase your folic acid intake through dietary sources. Some excellent foods rich in folate include:

1. Leafy Greens

Spinach, kale, and romaine lettuce are excellent sources of folate, a vital B-vitamin that plays a crucial role in cell growth and repair, making it especially important for pregnant women and those planning to conceive. Folate helps in the production of red blood cells and supports the healthy development of the neural tube in embryos, preventing certain birth defects.

2. Legumes

Beans, lentils, and chickpeas are not only rich in folate but also provide protein and fiber, which are beneficial during pregnancy.

3. Citrus Fruits

Oranges, grapefruits, and lemons are excellent sources of vitamin C and folate. Enjoy them as snacks or in juices.

4. Fortified Cereals

Many breakfast cereals are fortified with folic acid, making them an easy option for your morning meal.

5. Nuts and Seeds

Almonds and sunflower seeds can add a folate boost to your diet. They also provide healthy fats and protein.

Incorporating a variety of these foods into your meals can help ensure you meet your folic acid needs during pregnancy.

Iron: Supporting Blood Health and Development

Iron is another essential nutrient that plays a critical role during pregnancy. Your body requires more iron to support the increased blood volume that comes with pregnancy. Iron helps produce hemoglobin, the protein in red blood cells that carries oxygen to your baby. An adequate intake of iron is essential to prevent iron-deficiency anemia, which can lead to fatigue, weakness, and complications during delivery.

During pregnancy, you need approximately 27 milligrams of iron daily, which is significantly higher than the amount needed when you're not pregnant. This increase is necessary to ensure your body can supply enough oxygen to both you and your growing baby.

Sources of Iron

To meet your iron needs, focus on both heme iron (found in animal products) and non-heme iron (found in plant-based foods). Your body absorbes heme iron more easily. Here are some excellent sources of iron:

1. Lean Meats

Beef, chicken, and turkey are excellent sources of heme iron, a type of iron that is particularly well-absorbed by the body compared to non-heme iron, which is found in plant-based foods. Consider adding lean cuts of meat to your meals a few times a week.

2. Fish

Fatty fish like salmon not only provide iron but also omega-3 fatty acids, which are beneficial for your baby's brain development.

3. Legumes

Beans, lentils, and chickpeas are rich in non-heme iron. They also offer protein and fiber, making them excellent choices for pregnant women.

4. Tofu

This plant-based protein is a versatile option that can easily be incorporated into stir-fries and salads, providing both protein and iron.

5. Dark Chocolate

A delicious way to boost your iron intake, dark chocolate (with a cocoa content of 70% or higher) can be enjoyed in moderation as a treat.

6. Nuts and Seeds

Pumpkin seeds, sunflower seeds, and cashews are not only great snacks but also good sources of non-heme iron.

To enhance iron absorption from non-heme sources, pair these foods with vitamin C-rich options. For instance, enjoy a salad with chickpeas and add some sliced bell peppers or oranges for a nutrient boost.

When to Consider Supplements

While it's best to get your nutrients from food, sometimes dietary sources alone aren't enough, especially when it comes to folic acid and iron. If you're struggling to meet your needs through diet or if your healthcare provider identifies a deficiency, they may recommend supplements.

Taking a prenatal vitamin that includes both folic acid and iron can help ensure you're getting the right amounts. Always consult with your healthcare provider before starting any new supplements, as they can help determine the right dosage for you.

Monitoring Your Levels

As your pregnancy progresses, your healthcare provider will likely monitor your iron and folate levels through routine blood tests. If you're found to be deficient in either nutrient, they will provide recommendations on dietary changes and supplementation to help improve your levels. It's essential to stay on top of these check-ups to ensure both your health and your baby's development.

Strategic Suggestions

- **Incorporate a variety of folate-rich foods** like leafy greens, legumes, and fortified cereals into your meals.

- **Aim for iron-rich sources** such as lean meats, fish, and legumes, and combine them with vitamin C to boost absorption.

- **Take prenatal vitamins** that include adequate amounts of folic acid and iron if your diet isn't meeting your needs.

- **Monitor your levels through regular check-ups** to ensure you're getting enough of these essential nutrients.

- **Consider cooking in cast iron pots and pans**, which can increase the iron content of your food.

Folic acid and iron are critical during the first trimester, and understanding their roles will help you make informed dietary choices. Focus on a balanced diet rich in these nutrients to

support both your health and your baby's
development during this crucial time.

Managing Fatigue with Proper Diet

Fatigue is one of the most common complaints during the first trimester of pregnancy, often making everyday tasks feel overwhelming. Hormonal changes, increased blood volume, and the body's energy demands all contribute to that tired feeling. However, what you eat can play a major role in managing fatigue. Choosing the right foods and maintaining steady energy levels throughout the day can help you feel more energized and keep you from becoming overly exhausted.

Understanding the Causes of Fatigue in Pregnancy

In the first trimester, your body is working hard to support the growth and development of your baby. This increased demand on your body's energy reserves, along with hormonal changes (especially the rise in progesterone), can leave you feeling drained. Progesterone, while essential for maintaining pregnancy, has a calming effect on the body, which can also lead to feelings of tiredness.

The changes in blood volume during pregnancy also contribute to fatigue. As your body produces more blood to supply oxygen to your growing baby, your heart works harder, and you may feel more tired. In addition, your blood sugar levels may fluctuate, causing energy dips and making it difficult to stay awake and alert.

While fatigue is a normal part of pregnancy, there are things you can do to manage it through your diet and lifestyle choices. Fueling your body with the right nutrients can help provide sustained energy and prevent energy crashes.

Foods to Boost Your Energy

Eating nutrient-dense foods at regular intervals can help keep your energy levels stable throughout the day. A well-balanced diet provides the nutrients needed to support your pregnancy while helping to avoid the dips and spikes in blood sugar that can lead to tiredness.

Complex Carbohydrates for Steady Energy

Carbohydrates are the body's main source of energy. During pregnancy, it's especially important to choose complex carbohydrates, which provide a steady release of energy over time. Foods like whole grains (brown rice, whole wheat bread, oats, quinoa) and starchy vegetables (sweet potatoes, squash) are excellent choices. These foods have a low glycemic index, meaning they don't cause a rapid spike in blood sugar and can help prevent the energy crashes that can leave you feeling fatigued.

Protein to Maintain Strength

Protein is crucial during pregnancy as it helps support the development of your baby's tissues, as well as your own muscle and immune systems. Eating adequate amounts of protein at each meal can help stabilize your blood sugar levels, keeping your energy steady. Good sources of protein include lean meats like chicken or turkey, fish (rich in omega-3 fatty acids), eggs, beans, lentils, tofu, and nuts.

Iron-Rich Foods to Prevent Fatigue

As discussed earlier, iron is essential for the production of hemoglobin, which carries oxygen in the blood. When you don't have enough iron, you may experience fatigue, dizziness, or weakness. Incorporating iron-rich foods into your diet can help prevent iron-deficiency anemia, which is a common cause of fatigue during pregnancy. Lean meats, leafy greens, beans, and fortified cereals are all great sources of iron. Pairing iron-rich foods with vitamin C—found in citrus fruits, bell peppers, and tomatoes—can enhance iron absorption.

Healthy Fats for Sustained Energy

Healthy fats, such as those found in avocados, olive oil, nuts, and seeds, are essential for maintaining your energy levels. These fats provide a steady, slow-burning source of energy and help with the absorption of fat-soluble vitamins like A, D, E, and K. Omega-3 fatty acids, in particular, support brain function and development for both you and your baby. Including these healthy fats in your diet can help you avoid feelings of sluggishness and keep you feeling energized.

Hydration for Vitality

Dehydration can also contribute to fatigue, so it's important to drink plenty of fluids throughout the day. When you're pregnant, your body's fluid needs increase, and not getting enough water can make you feel more tired. Aim to drink at least 8-10 cups of water daily. You can also hydrate with herbal teas, coconut water, and fresh fruit or vegetable juices. Avoid sugary drinks, as they can cause a rapid rise in blood sugar, then a sharp drop, leaving you feeling more tired.

Meal Timing for Consistent Energy

In addition to choosing the right foods, when you eat them also matters. Eating smaller meals more frequently throughout the day can help maintain your energy levels. Instead of relying on three large meals, aim to have five or six smaller meals. This approach helps stabilize your blood sugar levels and prevents energy dips.

- **Breakfast**

Start your day with a balanced breakfast that includes complex carbs, protein, and healthy fats. A whole grain toast with avocado and a boiled egg, or oatmeal with chia seeds and fruit, can provide a great combination to fuel your day.

- **Mid-morning snack**

A handful of nuts, a piece of fruit, or a small yogurt can be excellent, quick snacks that provide an instant energy boost while also offering a range of essential nutrients.

- **Lunch and Dinner**

Both should focus on a balanced plate—protein, complex carbs, and vegetables. A quinoa salad with chicken, beans, and a variety of colorful vegetables is a great choice.

- **Afternoon snack**

Another small snack, like a piece of dark chocolate with almonds, can help keep your energy up during the late afternoon slump.

Other Tips for Managing Fatigue

While food plays a crucial role in managing fatigue, there are other lifestyle factors that can make a difference as well:

- **Rest when you can**

Listening to your body and allowing yourself to rest when needed is crucial for both your physical and mental well-being. In our fast-paced world, it's easy to fall into the trap of pushing through fatigue, stress, or discomfort.

Take naps or simply sit down with your feet up if you feel tired.

- **Gentle exercise**

If you're able, try light physical activity like walking or prenatal yoga. Exercise can help improve circulation and boost your energy levels.

- **Good sleep hygiene**

Aim for 7-9 hours of sleep each night. Try to establish a bedtime routine and avoid caffeine late in the day to ensure you get a restful night's sleep.

Strategic Suggestions

- **Focus on whole grains** like brown rice, oats, and quinoa for sustained energy throughout the day.
- **Incorporate iron-rich foods** like leafy greens, beans, and lean meats to prevent anemia-related fatigue.

- **Consume healthy fats** from sources like avocados, olive oil, and nuts to maintain energy and absorb key vitamins.
- **Stay hydrated** with water, herbal teas, and fresh juices to avoid dehydration and boost energy.
- **Eat small, balanced meals regularly** to maintain stable blood sugar and prevent energy crashes.

Fatigue is a normal part of pregnancy, but with the right dietary choices and lifestyle adjustments, you can manage it effectively. Focusing on a balanced diet, staying hydrated, and ensuring you're getting the right nutrients at the right times will help you feel more energized and ready to take on the demands of the first trimester.

Chapter 3: Second Trimester Nutrition

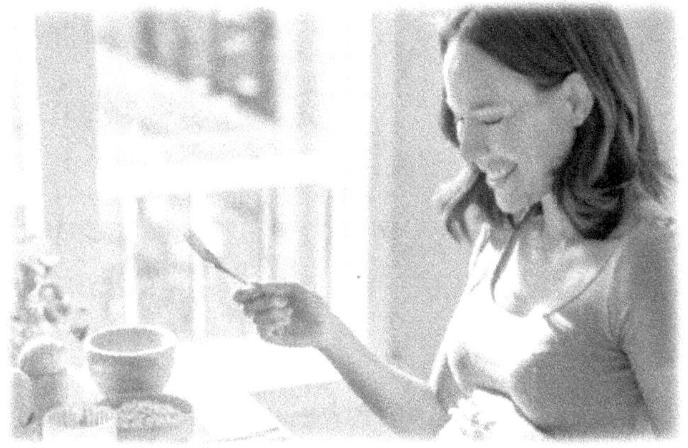

Second Trimester Nutrition is crucial as it marks a period of significant growth for both you and your baby. During this phase, your nutritional needs increase to support developing organs, bones, and muscles. A well-balanced diet ensures optimal health and sets the foundation for a healthy pregnancy.

Growing Baby, Growing Appetite: Eating for Two

As you enter the second trimester, your body undergoes some exciting changes. Your baby is growing rapidly, and with that growth comes an increased appetite. It's common for expectant mothers to feel hungrier than usual during this time, and it's important to understand why. In this phase, your body needs more nutrients to support both your baby's development and your own energy needs. But eating for two doesn't necessarily mean doubling your food intake. Instead, it's about making smarter, more nutritious food choices to nourish both you and your baby.

Why Appetite Increases in the Second Trimester

During the second trimester, your baby is growing quickly. By the end of this trimester, your baby's organs and systems are beginning to function more fully. The placenta, which provides oxygen and nutrients to your baby, is growing as well, increasing your nutritional demands. As your baby develops, your metabolism speeds up, requiring more energy from food.

While you don't need to double the amount of food you're eating, it's essential to increase the quality of your meals and focus on nutrient-dense foods. A healthy and balanced diet will ensure that both you and your baby receive the vitamins, minerals, and energy needed for healthy growth and development. In this phase, your increased appetite is a natural response to the body's demands for more calories, protein, and other essential nutrients.

Meeting the Nutritional Demands of the Second Trimester

In the second trimester, you should aim to eat around 300 extra calories per day. These extra calories don't mean indulging in empty calories from sugary snacks or processed foods. Instead, they should come from nutrient-rich, whole foods that provide the necessary vitamins, minerals, and proteins for both you and your growing baby.

Here are the key nutrients you should focus on during this stage:

1. Protein for Growth

Protein is essential for the growth of your baby's cells and tissues. It also helps with the production of amniotic fluid and supports the development of your placenta. Good sources of protein include lean meats like chicken and turkey, fish, eggs, dairy products, legumes like beans and lentils, and plant-based options like tofu and tempeh.

2. Complex Carbohydrates for Energy

Your growing baby needs energy, and complex carbohydrates are your body's primary source. These provide a steady release of energy to keep you going throughout the day. Choose whole grains like brown rice, oats, quinoa, and whole wheat bread. Sweet potatoes, butternut squash, and other starchy vegetables also provide valuable carbs.

3. Healthy Fats for Brain Development

Healthy fats, especially omega-3 fatty acids, play a crucial role in your baby's brain and eye development. Fatty fish like salmon, chia seeds, flaxseeds, and walnuts are excellent sources of omega-3s. You should also include other healthy fats, such as those found in avocados, olive oil, and nuts, to help keep your energy levels up and support the absorption of fat-soluble vitamins like A, D, E, and K.

4. Fruits and Vegetables for Vitamins and Fiber

Fruits and vegetables are rich in vitamins, minerals, and antioxidants that help both you and your baby stay healthy. They are also an excellent source of fiber, which helps prevent constipation, a common issue during pregnancy. Aim for a variety of colorful fruits and veggies—leafy greens like spinach and kale, berries, oranges, carrots, and bell peppers provide a range of nutrients, including folate, vitamin C, and fiber.

5. Calcium and Vitamin D for Bone Health

Both calcium and vitamin D are crucial for building your baby's bones and teeth. Dairy products like milk, yogurt, and cheese are excellent sources of calcium, while fortified plant-based milks (such as almond or soy milk) also provide calcium. Vitamin D, which helps your body absorb calcium, is found in fortified foods, fatty fish like salmon, and can also be synthesized by your body with exposure to sunlight.

Eating Smarter, Not More

It's tempting to think that eating for two means eating double the portion size, but it's important to remember that quality matters more than quantity. Your body needs more nutrients, not more food. Here are some practical tips to ensure you're meeting your increased nutritional needs without overeating:

- **Focus on nutrient-dense snacks**

Instead of reaching for empty-calorie snacks like chips or cookies, try snacking on foods that provide nutrients, such as yogurt with fruit, a handful of nuts, or sliced vegetables with hummus. These snacks will help keep you full and provide essential vitamins and minerals.

- **Use smaller, balanced meals**

Eating smaller, more frequent meals throughout the day can help manage your appetite and maintain steady energy levels. Aim for 5-6 meals, including a combination of protein, healthy fats, and whole grains to keep you feeling satisfied longer.

- **Stay hydrated**

Dehydration can sometimes be mistaken for hunger. Make sure to drink plenty of water throughout the day, especially as your body's fluid needs increase during pregnancy. Herbal teas and fresh juices are great ways to hydrate as well.

- **Include a variety of food groups**

A diverse diet will ensure that you're getting a wide range of nutrients. Include lean proteins, whole grains, fruits, vegetables, and healthy fats in every meal. Try to eat the rainbow, choosing colorful fruits and vegetables to get a variety of vitamins and minerals.

- **Listen to your body**

Pregnancy is a time when your body may go through fluctuations in appetite. Some days you may feel hungrier than others, and that's okay. The key is to eat when you're hungry and focus on nutrient-rich foods.

Strategic Suggestions

- **Increase protein intake** through lean meats, legumes, tofu, and dairy products to support your baby's growth.

- **Focus on whole grains and healthy carbs** like oats, quinoa, and sweet potatoes to provide long-lasting energy.
- **Include healthy fats** like omega-3s from fish, walnuts, and chia seeds to support brain development.
- **Snack wisely on nutrient-dense options** like yogurt with fruit, nuts, or veggie sticks with hummus.
- Stay hydrated with water, herbal teas, and fresh juices to support increased fluid needs.

Eating well during the second trimester is about nourishing your body and supporting your baby's rapid growth. Focus on nutrient-rich, whole foods and listen to your body's cues to meet your increased energy needs without overindulging. It's not about eating for two in the traditional sense, but about making every bite count for both you and your baby's health.

Calcium and Vitamin D: Building Strong Bones and Teeth

Calcium and vitamin D are two essential nutrients that play a critical role in your pregnancy, particularly as your baby's bones and teeth begin to develop. During the second trimester, your baby's skeleton is growing at a fast pace, and both calcium and vitamin D are necessary for bone mineralization and overall health. Getting enough of these nutrients is also important for you, as they help maintain your bone density and prevent issues like muscle cramps and bone loss during pregnancy.

Why Calcium and Vitamin D Matter During Pregnancy

Calcium is a vital mineral for both you and your baby. During pregnancy, it helps form your baby's bones, teeth, and nervous system. Calcium is also crucial for maintaining your bone health. As your baby's skeleton forms, your body will use a large portion of the calcium it takes in to ensure proper bone development. To meet the baby's growing needs, your body draws calcium from your bones, which means it's important for you to have a good intake of calcium to help prevent any depletion in your own bones. Without enough calcium, you could be at higher risk of developing pregnancy-related complications, like preeclampsia, or suffer from leg cramps, muscle weakness, and bone pain.

Vitamin D plays a complementary role to calcium. It helps your body absorb calcium more efficiently and supports the development of your baby's bones and immune system. Without enough vitamin D, your body might not absorb enough calcium, even if you're consuming adequate amounts. This can lead to weaker bones, not just for your baby, but for you as well. Vitamin D also helps reduce the risk of conditions like osteoporosis, which can cause fragile bones later in life.

Both nutrients are crucial for the overall health of your pregnancy, and the second trimester is a key time to ensure you're getting enough to support your baby's rapid development.

How Much Calcium and Vitamin D Do You Need?

During the second trimester, your body needs more calcium than it did during the first trimester, as your baby's bones and teeth are growing rapidly. Most pregnant women need about 1,000 milligrams of calcium per day. This increases to 1,200 milligrams per day if you are under 19 years old. The Recommended Dietary Allowance (RDA) for vitamin D is 600 IU (International Units) per day during pregnancy. This number may vary based on your geographical location, sun exposure, and other factors, but maintaining an intake of at least 600 IU is generally recommended.

If you are not getting enough from your diet or from the sun, you might need a supplement. Consult your healthcare provider to determine the right amount of vitamin D for you, especially if you have risk factors like a history of osteoporosis, limited sun exposure, or darker skin, which can make it harder to produce vitamin D naturally.

Best Food Sources of Calcium and Vitamin D

Getting calcium and vitamin D from food sources is the best way to ensure you're getting these nutrients in the correct amounts. Here's a list of foods rich in each:

Calcium-Rich Foods:

- **Dairy Products:** Milk, yogurt, and cheese are the most well-known sources of calcium. A cup of milk or yogurt typically contains around 300 milligrams of calcium. Cheese, particularly hard cheeses like cheddar, also pack a punch with calcium.

- **Leafy Greens:** Vegetables like kale, collard greens, and spinach are rich in calcium. However, spinach also contains oxalates, which can interfere with calcium absorption, so try to focus on other greens like kale and collard greens.

- **Fortified Foods:** Many plant-based milks (such as almond milk, soy milk, and oat milk) are fortified with calcium. Check the label to make sure they contain calcium.

- **Tofu and Tempeh:** These plant-based protein sources are also high in calcium, especially when made with calcium sulfate. Tofu can be added to stir-fries, soups, and smoothies for an easy calcium boost.

- **Beans and Lentils:** White beans, chickpeas, and lentils contain moderate amounts of calcium, along with fiber and protein.

Vitamin D-Rich Foods:

- **Fatty Fish:** Fish like salmon, mackerel, and sardines are excellent sources of vitamin D. A 3-ounce serving of salmon provides around 570 IU of vitamin D, which is nearly the full daily recommended amount.

- **Egg Yolks:** Eggs contain small amounts of vitamin D, particularly in the yolks. Add a couple of eggs to your breakfast or incorporate them into your meals to get some extra vitamin D.

- **Fortified Foods:** Like calcium, vitamin D is often added to plant-based milks (soy, almond, or oat milk), breakfast cereals, and some brands of orange juice. When buying fortified products, always check the labels to ensure they contain adequate levels of vitamin D.

- **Mushrooms:** Certain varieties of mushrooms, such as maitake and shiitake, contain small amounts of vitamin D, especially when they have been exposed to UV light. Consider adding them to your meals for a plant-based source of this vitamin.

The Role of Sunlight in Vitamin D Production

Your body naturally produces vitamin D when your skin is exposed to sunlight. However, many factors can influence your body's ability to make vitamin D from sunlight, such as living in areas with limited sunlight, especially during the winter months, or having darker skin, which requires more sunlight to produce the same amount of vitamin D. Vitamin D plays a vital role in supporting overall health, yet many people may not be getting enough of it, particularly if they live in regions with limited sunlight or have lifestyles that prevent adequate sun exposure.

Managing Deficiency

If you are found to have a deficiency in calcium or vitamin D, your healthcare provider may recommend supplements. It's important not to self-prescribe these, as taking too much of either nutrient can have adverse effects. A calcium supplement can cause constipation, while too much vitamin D can lead to calcium build-up in the blood, which can be harmful to your organs.

Strategic Suggestions

- **Consume dairy or fortified plant-based alternatives** like almond or soy milk to boost calcium intake.
- **Incorporate fatty fish** such as salmon, sardines, or mackerel into meals for a good dose of vitamin D.
- **Snack on calcium-rich foods** like cheese, yogurt, or fortified cereals.
- **Add leafy greens** like kale, collard greens, and broccoli to your meals to increase calcium intake naturally.
- **Aim for sunlight exposure** whenever possible to help your body produce vitamin D naturally.

Incorporating calcium and vitamin D into your daily routine is vital for your health and your baby's development. These nutrients are key in building strong bones and teeth and ensuring that both you and your baby thrive throughout the pregnancy. Eat a balanced diet, get some sun, and make sure you meet your nutritional need to set both of you up for a healthy and strong future.

Protein Needs for Baby's Development

Protein is one of the most important nutrients during pregnancy. As you enter the second trimester, your body's need for protein increases significantly to support your growing baby's rapid development. Protein plays a vital role in building and repairing tissues, producing enzymes and hormones, and supporting your baby's overall growth, particularly as organs, muscles, and the brain begin to form.

Why Protein is Essential for Baby's Development

Protein is a key building block for your baby's development. During the second trimester, your baby is developing more rapidly than before, and this is when the creation of bones, muscles, and organs takes off. Protein provides the amino acids that are essential for these processes. Your baby's cells are constantly dividing, and protein is crucial for creating these new cells.

Along with supporting the baby's growth, protein is also necessary for maintaining your own bodily functions during pregnancy. As your body adapts to the changes, you need more protein to help support the increased blood volume, your expanding uterus, and the growth of your placenta. Protein also helps in the production of breast tissue in preparation for breastfeeding after birth. It's important to remember that this nutrient doesn't just help the baby directly; it also keeps you feeling strong and energized throughout the day.

How Much Protein Do You Need During Pregnancy?

During pregnancy, especially in the second trimester, your body requires more protein than usual. While the general recommendation is about 46 grams of protein per day for a non-pregnant woman, pregnant women need more. In the second trimester, the recommendation increases to 71 grams of protein per day. This is an important target to meet to ensure your baby's growth and to keep your energy levels stable.

If you're carrying multiples (twins or more), you may need even more protein. However, it's always best to consult with your healthcare provider to assess your individual needs based on your health and pregnancy.

Best Sources of Protein

There are many delicious and nutritious protein-rich foods you can include in your diet to meet your daily needs. Here are some of the best sources:

1. Lean Meats

Lean cuts of beef, chicken, turkey, and pork are not only delicious but also outstanding sources of high-quality protein, making them an essential part of a balanced and nutritious diet. They also provide important nutrients like iron and zinc, which are essential during pregnancy.

A 3-ounce serving of lean meat contains around 20-30 grams of protein.

2. Fish

Fish is another great protein source, but it's important to choose low-mercury options like salmon, tilapia, and cod. Fatty fish like salmon is especially beneficial because it's high in omega-3 fatty acids, which are important for your baby's brain development. Avoid fish high in mercury, like swordfish and king mackerel, as too much mercury can be harmful.

3. Eggs

Eggs are a fantastic source of protein and other essential nutrients like choline, which supports your baby's brain development. One large egg provides about 6 grams of protein, and they can be easily added to various meals. Eggs are also versatile, and you can enjoy them scrambled, hard-boiled, or poached.

4. Legumes

Beans, lentils, chickpeas, and other legumes are excellent plant-based sources of protein. They're also rich in fiber, iron, and folate, which are important for your health and your baby's development. A cup of cooked lentils contains about 18 grams of protein. They can be incorporated into soups, stews, and salads or used as a meat substitute in various dishes.

5. Dairy Products

Dairy products like milk, yogurt, and cheese are not only rich in calcium but also provide a good amount of protein. A cup of Greek yogurt, for example, contains around 10-20 grams of protein. Opt for low-fat or fat-free versions if you're concerned about extra calories, but full-fat dairy can be a healthy choice in moderation.

6. Tofu and Tempeh

If you follow a plant-based or vegetarian diet, tofu and tempeh are excellent sources of protein. Tofu provides around 10 grams of protein per half-cup serving, and tempeh provides about 15 grams per half-cup serving. Both are incredibly versatile and can be used in stir-fries, salads, or even smoothies.

7. Nuts and Seeds

Almonds, peanuts, chia seeds, and hemp seeds are great sources of plant-based protein and healthy fats. A small handful of almonds (about 23 nuts) contains around 6 grams of protein. You can snack on them or add them to yogurt, smoothies, or oatmeal for a protein boost.

8. Quinoa

Quinoa is a complete protein, meaning it contains all nine essential amino acids. A cup of cooked quinoa contains around 8 grams of protein. It's a great gluten-free alternative to rice or pasta and can be added to salads, grain bowls, or even as a base for stir-fries.

Balancing Protein with Other Nutrients

While protein is crucial, it's important to balance it with other nutrients to create a well-rounded diet. In addition to protein, ensure you are consuming adequate amounts of vitamins, minerals, healthy fats, and fiber. Eating a variety of food groups ensures that you and your baby get the full spectrum of nutrients you need for health and development.

Protein and Hydration

Eating more protein may also require you to drink more water. As your body works to digest and metabolize higher amounts of protein, it needs adequate hydration. Staying well-hydrated will also help prevent common pregnancy discomforts like constipation and leg cramps, which dehydration aggravates. Aim to drink plenty of water throughout the day.

Strategic Suggestions

- **Incorporate lean meats** like chicken, turkey, and lean beef into your meals to boost your protein intake.

- **Add fish like salmon or tilapia** to your diet, making sure to choose low-mercury options.

- **Snack on protein-rich foods** like hard-boiled eggs, nuts, and seeds for an easy protein boost.

- **Include legumes** such as beans, lentils, and chickpeas in soups, stews, and salads to increase protein and fiber intake.

- **Consider plant-based proteins** like tofu, tempeh, and quinoa, especially if you follow a vegetarian or vegan diet.

- **Stay hydrated with plenty of water** to help your body process the increased protein intake.

Protein is a key nutrient for both you and your baby during pregnancy. Make mindful choices and focus on nutrient-rich protein sources to ensure that both you and your baby are getting the support you need for healthy growth and development.

Chapter 4: Third Trimester Diet: Preparing for Birth

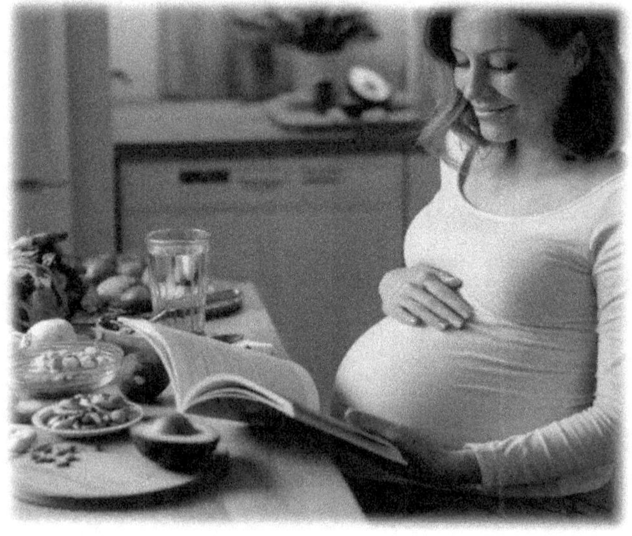

The third trimester is a critical period of growth and development for both mother and baby. Proper nutrition during these final months ensures optimal fetal health, supports maternal well-being, and prepares the body for labor. Focused dietary choices now can have lasting impacts on delivery and postpartum recovery.

Energy Requirements in the Final Stretch

As you approach the final stretch of your pregnancy, your body is working harder than ever to support both you and your baby. In the third trimester, your energy needs significantly increase. Your baby is growing rapidly, gaining weight, and developing crucial systems, while your body prepares for labor and delivery. Proper nutrition and adequate energy intake are essential for making sure you can keep up with these demands, maintain your strength, and support your baby's growth.

Understanding Increased Energy Needs

During the third trimester, the calorie requirement for most pregnant women increases 300 to 500 extra calories per day. This is due to the growing size of your baby, the rapid development of their organs and tissues, and the changes happening in your body to prepare for birth. These extra calories are vital to help you meet the demands of pregnancy and to provide the energy needed for daily activities.

It's important to note that these additional calories don't come from junk food or empty calories. Focus on nutrient-dense foods that provide essential vitamins, minerals, and macronutrients like protein, fiber, and healthy fats. The goal is to fuel your body with the right kind of energy—quality energy—not just more food.

What Happens to Your Energy Needs in the Third Trimester?

Your baby's growth is at its peak during this stage. By the end of the third trimester, your baby's weight can increase significantly, sometimes reaching 5 to 6 pounds or more. The baby's bones are hardening, muscles are building, and the nervous system is rapidly developing. At the same time, your body is also getting ready for labor, which takes a lot of energy. Your uterus is expanding, your blood volume has increased, and you're storing energy in the form of fat to help with lactation after birth.

To meet these higher energy demands, your body taps into your fat stores, especially during the later part of pregnancy. However, you must replenish these stores regularly with the right foods to ensure that you have enough energy to support both yourself and your growing baby.

During the third trimester, fatigue can become a common issue. This could be a result of the physical strain of carrying extra weight, as well as the hormonal changes that occur. Keeping your energy levels stable will help you feel more energized throughout the day and prepare for the challenges of labor.

How to Meet the Increased Energy Needs

To keep your energy levels up in the final trimester, make sure you're eating regularly throughout the day and choosing nutrient-rich foods that fuel both you and your baby. Here are some strategies to help you meet your increased energy needs:

1. Focus on Whole Grains

Foods like brown rice, whole wheat bread, quinoa, and oatmeal are rich in complex carbohydrates, which provide a steady, slow-releasing source of energy. These foods also contain fiber, which will help prevent constipation, a common issue during pregnancy. Whole grains can give you long-lasting energy without the blood sugar spikes and crashes that come from refined carbohydrates, like white bread or sugary snacks.

2. Prioritize Protein

Protein is not only important for your baby's growth but also helps maintain your muscle mass, prevent hunger pangs, and stabilize your blood sugar levels. Include protein-rich foods such as lean meats, poultry, fish, eggs, tofu, beans, and legumes in every meal. Protein helps build and repair tissues, so your body will need it as it adjusts for the birth process. Aim for about 71 grams of protein per day during the third trimester.

3. Healthy Fats for Extra Energy

Fats are an excellent source of concentrated energy. Healthy fats from sources like avocados, nuts, seeds, olive oil, and fatty fish (like salmon) provide a steady energy source. Omega-3 fatty acids, found in fatty fish and some plant-based oils, are also important for your baby's brain development, so don't shy away from these healthy fats. Just be mindful of portion sizes, as fats are calorie-dense.

4. Small, Frequent Meals

If you're finding it difficult to eat large meals due to the baby pressing on your stomach, try eating smaller, more frequent meals throughout the day. Snack on nutrient-dense foods such as Greek yogurt, hard-boiled eggs, or whole grain crackers with cheese. Eating regularly ensures that you're providing a steady supply of energy for your body and baby. Keep healthy snacks in your bag or kitchen so you can grab something whenever you're hungry.

5. Stay Hydrated

Staying hydrated is crucial during pregnancy, particularly in the third trimester, when your body is working harder to support both you and your baby. Proper hydration helps with digestion, circulation, and energy levels. Drink plenty of water throughout the day, and add water-rich foods like fruits (watermelon, oranges) and vegetables (cucumbers, lettuce) to your meals. Dehydration can make you feel sluggish and tired, so make sure to sip on water consistently throughout the day.

6. Avoid Empty Calories

Although you may feel the temptation to indulge in extra sweets or processed snacks, they don't provide the sustained energy your body needs. Try to avoid sugary snacks, junk food, or foods that provide empty calories, as they can lead to energy crashes and don't support the healthy growth of your baby. Focus on whole, nutrient-dense foods that provide vitamins, minerals, and fiber along with your extra calories.

Managing Energy Levels with Sleep and Rest

Along with a balanced diet, it's important to get enough rest in the third trimester. You may feel increasingly fatigued as your body prepares for labor, and taking the time to rest can help you recharge. Consider taking naps during the day if you're feeling tired, and aim for 7-9 hours of sleep each night. Proper sleep helps your body recover and ensures that you have the energy needed for both the physical demands of pregnancy and for the arrival of your baby.

Strategic Suggestions

- **Choose complex carbs** like whole grains to provide long-lasting energy without blood sugar spikes.

- **Incorporate lean protein** at each meal to support muscle mass, stabilize blood sugar, and curb hunger.

- **Include healthy fats** from sources like avocados, nuts, and fatty fish to fuel your body and your baby.

- **Snack frequently on nutritious foods** like yogurt, nuts, and fruits to maintain energy levels throughout the day.

- **Hydrate regularly** with water and water-rich foods like fruits and vegetables to prevent fatigue and support digestion.

- **Get adequate rest**, sleeping well at night and taking naps during the day to conserve energy.

In the final trimester, your body requires more fuel to support both you and your growing baby. Focus on nutrient-dense foods that provide quality energy, and remember to rest and stay hydrated. With the right approach, you'll have the strength and stamina to get through the last phase of pregnancy and prepare for the arrival of your baby.

Omega-3 Fatty Acids and Brain Development

During the third trimester of pregnancy, your baby's brain undergoes rapid growth and development. This period is crucial for setting the foundation for cognitive function and future learning abilities. One of the most important nutrients for supporting brain development during this time is omega-3 fatty acids, particularly DHA (docosahexaenoic acid). As an expecting mother, incorporating omega-3 fatty acids into your diet can have a profound impact on your baby's brain health and development.

Why Omega-3 Fatty Acids Matter

Omega-3 fatty acids are essential fats that play a vital role in the development of your baby's brain and nervous system. DHA, in particular, is a major component of the brain, making up a large part of the structure of brain cells. During the third trimester, your baby's brain is growing rapidly, and the omega-3s in your diet are used to form the neural connections that are critical for cognitive function, memory, and learning. DHA also contributes to the development of the retina, which is key for the baby's vision.

In fact, studies show that babies born to mothers who had adequate omega-3 levels during pregnancy tend to have better visual acuity and cognitive function later on. Proper omega-3 intake during pregnancy may even help reduce the risk of developmental delays, ADHD, and other neurological issues in childhood.

For you as an expectant mother, omega-3s also provide numerous benefits. They support your heart health, reduce inflammation, and may even help to ease pregnancy-related conditions like depression and anxiety. Omega-3s are known for their anti-inflammatory properties, which can help soothe aches and pains that come with pregnancy. Additionally, they can help regulate your mood and support mental well-being, which is especially important in the final stretch of pregnancy as you prepare for childbirth.

How Much Omega-3 Do You Need?

During pregnancy, particularly in the third trimester, you should aim to get around 200-300 mg of DHA per day. This amount supports your baby's brain development while helping to maintain your own health. Omega-3 fatty acids play a crucial role in overall health, and their importance during pregnancy cannot be overstated. Despite their numerous health benefits, many people don't consume enough omega-3s, which can be a significant concern for pregnant women.

While your body can make some omega-3s from other fats, it's important to get sufficient DHA from your diet to meet your baby's needs. Since omega-3s are primarily found in certain foods, you'll need to incorporate them regularly to ensure both you and your baby are getting the right amount.

Best Sources of Omega-3 Fatty Acids

The best sources of omega-3 fatty acids are fatty fish, but there are also plant-based sources available. Here are some top options to consider:

1. Fatty Fish

Fatty fish like salmon, mackerel, sardines, and trout are the richest sources of DHA. These fish are also high in EPA (eicosapentaenoic acid), another beneficial omega-3 fatty acid. Aim for at least 2-3 servings of fatty fish per week. A 3-ounce serving of salmon, for example, provides around 1,000 mg of DHA, which is more than enough to meet your daily needs.

2. Chia Seeds

If you follow a plant-based or vegetarian diet, chia seeds are an excellent source of omega-3s, although they provide ALA (alpha-linolenic acid), which needs to be converted into DHA in your body. Chia seeds contain around 5 grams of ALA per ounce. They can be sprinkled on oatmeal, added to smoothies, or mixed into baked goods.

3. Flaxseeds

Like chia seeds, flaxseeds are rich in ALA omega-3s. You can add ground flaxseeds to smoothies, yogurt, or cereals for a nutrient boost. One tablespoon of ground flaxseeds offers about 2.4 grams of ALA. Although it's plant-based, the conversion to DHA may not be as efficient as from fish sources, but it's still a good addition to your diet.

4. Walnuts

Walnuts are indeed one of the best plant-based sources of ALA (alpha-linolenic acid), a type of omega-3 fatty acid that is essential for health. A handful of walnuts (about 1 ounce or 14 halves) provides 2.5 grams of ALA (alpha-linolenic acid), making them one of the most potent plant-based sources of omega-3 fatty acids. They make a great snack on their own, or you can toss them into salads, yogurt, or oatmeal for added crunch and nutrition.

5. Algal Oil

Algal oil is derived from algae and is one of the few plant-based sources that contain DHA directly. It's a good option for vegetarians and vegans who want to ensure they're getting enough DHA without consuming fish. Algal oil supplements are available, and a typical dose provides around 200-300 mg of DHA per capsule, which can help you meet your needs.

6. Fortified Foods

Many foods are now fortified with omega-3s, including eggs, milk, and certain brands of yogurt or juices. These can be a convenient way to add extra DHA to your diet.

Additional Benefits of Omega-3s

Omega-3 fatty acids are not only important for brain development but also for overall pregnancy health. They have been linked to:

1. Reducing the risk of preterm labor

Omega-3s have anti-inflammatory properties that can help prevent premature contractions and support full-term pregnancy.

Reducing the risk of postpartum depression: Omega-3s play a role in regulating mood and emotions, which may help reduce the risk of postpartum depression.

2. Supporting heart health

Omega-3s are known for their cardiovascular benefits. During pregnancy, they help to reduce the risk of high blood pressure and preeclampsia, a pregnancy complication that affects the heart and blood vessels.

Strategic Suggestions

- **Incorporate fatty fish** like salmon, mackerel, and sardines into your meals 2-3 times a week to get your DHA from a reliable source.

- **Add chia seeds and flaxseeds** to your daily diet, using them in smoothies, cereals, or baked goods for an easy omega-3 boost.

- **Snack on walnuts or other nuts** rich in ALA to help support omega-3 intake throughout the day.

- **Consider algae-based DHA supplements** if you're not consuming enough omega-3s from fish or plant-based sources.

- **Choose fortified foods**, such as omega-3-enriched eggs, to further supplement your diet.

Incorporating omega-3s into your diet is an essential step in supporting your baby's brain development during the third trimester. It's a small adjustment that can have a big impact, both for your baby's health and for your own well-being. Aim for a combination of fish, plant-based sources, and supplements to make sure you're meeting your omega-3 needs for the final stretch of your pregnancy.

Hydration and Managing Common Third Trimester Symptoms

As you approach the final stretch of your pregnancy, staying hydrated becomes more important than ever. In the third trimester, your body's demands increase, and dehydration can lead to a number of uncomfortable symptoms, some of which are more pronounced as you near your due date. Maintaining proper hydration not only supports your overall health but also plays a key role in managing common third-trimester discomforts like swelling, constipation, fatigue, and even preterm labor.

Why Hydration Matters During the Third Trimester

Hydration is vital because your body is working overtime to support both you and your baby. In the third trimester, your blood volume increases, and your kidneys must work harder to filter out waste products. You are also producing more amniotic fluid, which cushions and protects your baby. Dehydration can have a direct impact on these processes, leading to complications such as high blood pressure, dizziness, constipation, and even contractions that may mimic preterm labor.

The need for water increases during pregnancy due to hormonal changes, the increase in blood volume, and the demands placed on your kidneys and circulatory system. As you approach delivery, dehydration can even increase the likelihood of complications such as a more prolonged labor or an increased risk of interventions like a C-section. Therefore, staying hydrated is key to your comfort and your baby's well-being in the final trimester.

How Much Water Do You Need?

Pregnancy generally requires about 10 cups (80 ounces) of fluids per day, but in the third trimester, you may need more, especially if you're experiencing symptoms like swelling or if you're more active. Some studies suggest pregnant women in the third trimester may need 12 cups of water daily to meet the demands of pregnancy.

It's essential to remember that the 10 cups should come from a combination of liquids—water, milk, and 100% fruit juice—along with high-water-content foods like fruits and vegetables. While water is the best option for hydration, you can also hydrate with foods such as watermelon, cucumbers, oranges, strawberries, and lettuce.

Hydration's Role in Managing Third Trimester Symptoms

1. Swelling (Edema)

One of the most common issues in the third trimester is swelling, particularly in the feet, ankles, and hands. This happens because your body retains extra fluid to accommodate the growing baby. Drinking enough water helps your kidneys function properly, and good kidney function ensures that the body can eliminate excess sodium and fluid, which can reduce swelling. Hydration also supports your circulatory system, helping blood flow more efficiently and preventing fluid from pooling in your lower extremities.

Practical Tip: Keep a water bottle with you throughout the day to remind yourself to sip regularly. You'll find that proper hydration can help alleviate the discomfort of swelling and keep you feeling more comfortable.

2. Constipation

Pregnancy hormones, particularly progesterone, slow down your digestive system, leading to constipation, a common issue in the third trimester. Inadequate hydration can worsen this condition because your body will draw water from the intestines to maintain hydration elsewhere, resulting in harder stools. Drinking plenty of water softens stools and helps keep everything moving smoothly.

Practical Tip: Along with drinking plenty of water, consider adding high-fiber foods like whole grains, vegetables, and fruits to your diet to ease constipation. Fiber helps bulk up stools, making them easier to pass.

3. Fatigue

Fatigue is common in the third trimester as your body works harder to support your baby. Dehydration can make this fatigue worse, leaving you feeling sluggish and drained. When you're dehydrated, your body has to work harder to maintain fluid balance, which can make you feel more tired.

Practical Tip: Aim to drink water throughout the day, especially if you're feeling tired. Sipping small amounts regularly rather than consuming large amounts all at once can be more effective. Try carrying a bottle with you to remind yourself to stay hydrated and boost your energy levels.

4. Preterm Labor

Dehydration has been associated with an increased risk of preterm labor. It can cause your uterus to contract prematurely. Staying hydrated can help reduce this risk, preventing unnecessary contractions and helping the body function efficiently as it prepares for labor.

Practical Tip: If you begin to experience signs of dehydration—such as dry mouth, dark yellow urine, or dizziness—take immediate steps to rehydrate, drinking water and consulting with your healthcare provider.

5. Breast Milk Production

Hydration is also important for postpartum health. Drinking enough water helps in the production of breast milk. After delivery, you'll need more fluids to produce milk and support breastfeeding, so staying hydrated in the third trimester is a great way to prepare your body for the postpartum period.

Tips for Staying Hydrated in the Third Trimester

1. Drink Water Consistently

Carry a water bottle with you at all times to make sure you're sipping water regularly. If plain water doesn't appeal to you, try infusing it with fruits like lemon, berries, or cucumber to make it more enjoyable.

2. Eat Hydrating Foods

Focus on eating water-rich foods like watermelon, cucumber, strawberries, and leafy greens. These can contribute to your hydration needs while providing additional vitamins and nutrients.

3. Limit Caffeine

Caffeine is a diuretic, meaning it can make you lose fluids more quickly. While it's okay to have an occasional cup of coffee or tea, try to limit your intake to prevent dehydration. Opt for caffeine-free herbal teas instead.

4. Avoid Sugary Drinks

Sugary sodas or juice drinks can lead to spikes in your blood sugar and don't hydrate you as effectively as water or natural fruit juices. Stick to healthier beverages that hydrate without the added sugars.

5. Stay Cool

During hot weather, you may lose more fluids through sweat. Be mindful to drink more water when the weather is warm or if you're more active.

6. Listen to Your Body

If you feel thirsty, don't ignore it. Thirst is a sign your body needs more hydration. Make sure to drink plenty of water if you feel parched or notice your urine becoming darker in color.

Strategic Suggestions

- **Aim for 10-12 cups of fluids daily**, primarily water, to maintain hydration levels.
- **Carry a water bottle with you** to remind yourself to drink throughout the day.

- **Incorporate hydrating foods** such as watermelon, cucumbers, and oranges into your meals.
- **Limit caffeine and sugary drinks**, opting instead for water or herbal teas.
- **Stay cool during hot days** and increase fluid intake when needed.

Maintaining proper hydration during the third trimester can alleviate common pregnancy discomforts like swelling, constipation, and fatigue. Drinking enough fluids to support your body's functions, reduce the risk of complications, and feel more energized as you prepare for labor and delivery. So, drink up—your body, and your baby, will thank you.

Chapter 5: Special Dietary Considerations for Pregnant Women

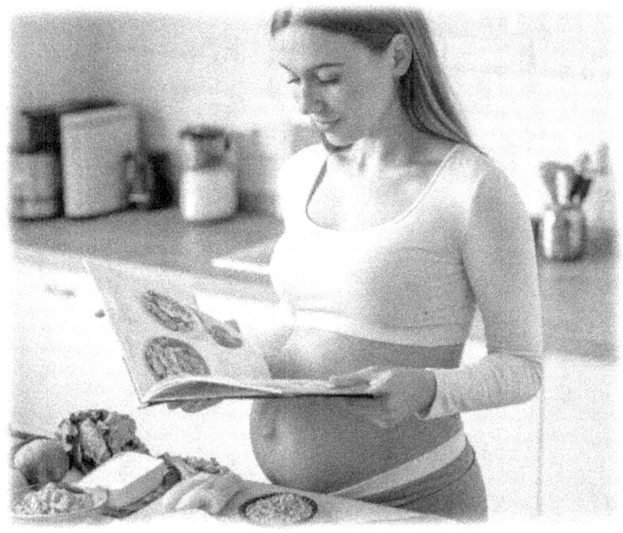

Special Dietary Considerations for Pregnant Women address the unique nutritional needs that arise due to medical conditions, food sensitivities, or lifestyle choices. Proper nutrition is essential during pregnancy, and adjusting your diet can help manage conditions like gestational diabetes, food allergies, and vegetarian or vegan diets for a healthy pregnancy.

Managing Gestational Diabetes with Diet

Gestational diabetes is a form of diabetes that develops during pregnancy. It typically occurs when the body cannot produce enough insulin to meet the increased needs during pregnancy, leading to higher blood sugar levels. Managing this condition with a balanced diet is crucial, as it helps control blood sugar levels and supports both your health and your baby's development.

Understanding Gestational Diabetes and Its Impact

When you're pregnant, your body undergoes many changes, including the increased production of pregnancy hormones like human placental lactogen, estrogen, and progesterone. These hormones can make your cells less responsive to insulin, a hormone that helps your body regulate blood sugar. As a result, your blood sugar levels may rise, leading to gestational diabetes.

Gestational diabetes can affect both you and your baby. If left unmanaged, it can increase the risk of complications such as excessive weight gain, preeclampsia, premature birth, and even stillbirth. Babies born to mothers with gestational diabetes are also at risk of being larger than average (macrosomia), which can lead to delivery complications and a higher likelihood of developing type 2 diabetes later in life.

The good news is that with careful management through diet, regular monitoring of blood sugar levels, and sometimes medication, gestational diabetes can be controlled, minimizing the risks to both you and your baby.

Dietary Strategies for Managing Gestational Diabetes

Managing gestational diabetes is largely about controlling blood sugar levels through a balanced, nutrient-dense diet. This means focusing on foods that release energy slowly and help keep your blood sugar levels stable. Here are some key strategies to consider:

1. Focus on Complex Carbohydrates

Carbohydrates are the body's main source of energy, but not all carbs are created equal. Simple carbohydrates—found in foods like white bread, pastries, and sugary drinks—are quickly absorbed into the bloodstream, leading to rapid spikes in blood sugar. Instead, opt for complex carbohydrates, which are digested more slowly and provide a more steady supply of energy.

- **Good options:** Whole grains like oats, brown rice, quinoa, and whole wheat bread. Also, legumes such as lentils and chickpeas provide fiber and protein along with carbs, which helps slow the absorption of sugar.

2. Choose High-Fiber Foods

Fiber plays a crucial role in controlling blood sugar. It slows down digestion and prevents blood sugar from spiking too quickly after meals. A diet rich in fiber will help keep your blood sugar levels stable and can also help prevent constipation, which is common during pregnancy.

- **Good options:** Vegetables (especially leafy greens), fruits (like berries and apples), beans, lentils, and whole grains. Aim to include a variety of these in your meals to ensure you're getting plenty of fiber.

3. Balance Your Meals with Lean Protein and Healthy Fats

Protein and healthy fats not only help keep you fuller longer but also slow down the absorption of sugars. A balanced meal with a mix of carbs, protein, and fat will ensure steady energy levels throughout the day.

- **Good protein options:** Lean meats (chicken, turkey), fish (especially those rich in omega-3s like salmon), eggs, tofu, and beans.

- **Healthy fats:** Avocados, nuts, seeds, and olive oil.

4. Monitor Portion Sizes

Even healthy foods can cause blood sugar levels to rise if eaten in large quantities. It's important to monitor portion sizes, especially when eating carbohydrate-rich foods. Spreading your meals throughout the day in smaller portions (e.g., three meals with two to three small snacks) can help stabilize blood sugar and prevent overeating at any one meal.

Practical tip: Use a small plate for meals and try to avoid second servings. This will help you stay mindful of your portion sizes.

5. Limit Sugary and Processed Foods

Foods that are high in refined sugars can cause rapid spikes in blood sugar. These include sugary drinks, candies, pastries, and other processed snacks. While occasional indulgence is fine, try to minimize your intake of these types of foods, especially since they don't provide the essential nutrients that both you and your baby need.

- **Healthy alternatives:** Opt for naturally sweet foods like fruits, which contain fiber along with natural sugars. You can also satisfy sweet cravings with dark chocolate (in moderation) or homemade energy bars made from oats and nuts.

6. Hydration is Key

Drinking plenty of water is essential for managing gestational diabetes. Staying hydrated helps your kidneys function properly, removing excess glucose from your bloodstream through urine. Additionally, proper hydration can prevent issues like fatigue, headaches, and leg cramps, which can be more common during pregnancy.

Practical tip: Aim to drink at least 8 cups of water daily. Carry a water bottle with you to ensure you're sipping throughout the day.

The Importance of Regular Monitoring

In addition to managing your diet, it's essential to regularly monitor your blood sugar levels to ensure they remain within a healthy range. Your doctor or healthcare provider will guide you on how often you should check your blood sugar and what your target levels should be.

Most women with gestational diabetes are advised to check their blood sugar levels at home multiple times a day, usually after meals. This helps you identify any foods or patterns that might be causing spikes in your blood sugar so you can adjust your diet as needed.

When Diet Alone Isn't Enough

For some women, diet alone may not be enough to control blood sugar levels, and insulin injections or oral medications might be prescribed. Insulin helps your body use glucose for energy, lowering blood sugar levels. If you're prescribed medication, it's important to follow your healthcare provider's instructions and keep track of your blood sugar levels to ensure the best outcomes.

Strategic Suggestions

- **Focus on complex carbs**, fiber-rich foods, and lean proteins to maintain steady blood sugar levels.

- **Avoid sugary and processed foods** that can cause rapid blood sugar spikes.

- **Monitor portion sizes** and aim for smaller, more frequent meals throughout the day.

- **Drink plenty of water to stay hydrated** to help maintain kidney function and overall health.

- **Regularly monitor blood sugar levels** and work closely with your healthcare provider to adjust your diet and treatment plan as needed.

Gestational diabetes can feel overwhelming, but with the right dietary adjustments and support from your healthcare team, you can manage the condition and enjoy a healthy pregnancy. A balanced diet will not only help regulate your blood sugar but also nourish you and your baby during this critical time.

Dealing with Food Allergies and Sensitivities

Food allergies and sensitivities can pose unique challenges during pregnancy, making it more important than ever to ensure that your diet meets both your nutritional needs and the safety of your baby. While pregnancy increases your body's demand for nutrients, certain foods may need to be avoided due to an allergy or intolerance. Understanding how to manage these food sensitivities while maintaining a balanced and nutritious diet will help you navigate your pregnancy with confidence.

Understanding Food Allergies and Sensitivities During Pregnancy

Food allergies occur when your immune system mistakenly identifies a typically harmless food as a threat. This results in an immune response that can cause symptoms ranging from mild discomfort, such as itching or hives, to more severe reactions, including anaphylaxis. Food sensitivities, on the other hand, are typically less severe and involve digestive issues, such as bloating or gas, rather than immune system involvement.

Common food allergies that can affect pregnant women include dairy, nuts, eggs, and seafood, while common sensitivities include gluten (in wheat and other grains) and lactose (in dairy products). For some women, pregnancy can also bring about new food sensitivities or even trigger a previously undiagnosed food allergy. This is due to changes in hormones and immune system function that occur during pregnancy, which can alter how your body reacts to different foods.

Food allergies and sensitivities can make it more difficult to get all the nutrients you need, so it's essential to manage your condition carefully while ensuring your body gets the vitamins, minerals, and protein it needs to support both your health and your baby's development.

Practical Ways to Manage Food Allergies and Sensitivities

If you have a food allergy or sensitivity, managing it during pregnancy involves more than simply avoiding problematic foods. You'll need to be proactive in ensuring your diet remains balanced and that you're meeting your nutritional needs.

1. Consult with Your Healthcare Provider

The first step in managing food allergies and sensitivities during pregnancy is to consult with your doctor or a registered dietitian. They can help you identify which foods should be avoided and suggest alternatives to ensure you're still getting all the necessary nutrients. Working with a healthcare professional will also ensure that your food choices are safe and aligned with your overall health goals.

2. Read Food Labels Carefully

Many packaged foods contain hidden ingredients that may be problematic for people with allergies or sensitivities. Common allergens like milk, eggs, soy, and nuts can be found in unexpected places, such as salad dressings, sauces, and packaged baked goods. Always read food labels carefully, and don't hesitate to contact manufacturers if you're unsure about the contents of a product.

3. Focus on a Diverse, Whole Food Diet

When dealing with food allergies and sensitivities, focusing on a whole food diet is key. This means choosing fresh fruits, vegetables, whole grains, lean proteins, and healthy fats, which are less likely to contain hidden allergens. A balanced, nutrient-rich diet will help you avoid allergens while ensuring you get the essential vitamins and minerals needed for a healthy pregnancy.

- **Good options for safe protein sources:** Chicken, turkey, fish (if not allergic), beans, lentils, and tofu (for those avoiding dairy or eggs).

- **Safe grains for gluten sensitivity:** Quinoa, rice, oats (ensure they are labeled gluten-free), and corn.

- **Dairy alternatives for those with lactose sensitivity or milk allergies:** Almond milk, coconut milk, or soy milk, as well as plant-based yogurts made from coconut or cashews.

4. Substitute Allergenic Foods with Nutrient-Rich Alternatives

For women with food allergies, finding safe alternatives is key to maintaining a balanced diet. For example, if you have a dairy allergy, you can switch to dairy-free alternatives like almond milk or soy yogurt. For those with nut allergies, try seeds like sunflower or chia, which provide similar nutritional benefits without the risk of an allergic reaction.

- **Egg-free baking:** Use flaxseed meal or chia seeds mixed with water as an egg replacement in baking. These alternatives are rich in omega-3 fatty acids and fiber.

- **Gluten-free options:** Many gluten-free breads and pastas are available today, but be mindful of their ingredients. Look for options made from rice, quinoa, or gluten-free oats, and ensure they are enriched with folic acid and iron, which are crucial during pregnancy.

5. Focus on Nutrients You May Be Missing

Depending on your allergies or sensitivities, you might need to pay extra attention to certain nutrients. For instance, if you avoid dairy due to a milk allergy or lactose intolerance, you might need to find alternative sources of calcium and vitamin D. If you're avoiding nuts due to an allergy, make sure you're getting healthy fats from other sources like avocados, seeds, and olive oil.

- **For calcium:** Leafy greens (such as kale and bok choy), fortified plant-based milks, tofu, and almonds (if not allergic).

- **For vitamin B12:** Fortified cereals, nutritional yeast, and certain plant-based milks can provide B12 if you are avoiding animal products or have sensitivities.

6. Maintain a Food Diary

Keeping a food diary is an excellent way to track what you're eating, how your body is reacting, and ensure you're avoiding trigger foods. This can be particularly helpful in identifying any new sensitivities or allergies that may emerge during pregnancy. It's also a useful tool for discussions with your healthcare provider or dietitian.

7. Consider Prenatal Vitamins

If you're struggling to meet all your nutritional needs due to food allergies or sensitivities, a prenatal vitamin can help fill in the gaps. Look for a supplement that contains essential nutrients like folic acid, calcium, iron, and omega-3s. Your doctor can recommend the best type of prenatal vitamin for your specific dietary needs.

Strategic Suggestions

- **Consult with a healthcare professional** to create a personalized dietary plan that ensures you avoid allergens while meeting your nutritional needs.

- **Read food labels thoroughly** to identify hidden allergens in processed foods.

- **Prioritize whole, unprocessed foods** like fresh fruits, vegetables, and lean proteins to minimize exposure to allergens.

- **Use allergen-free substitutes** for common allergens like dairy, eggs, and gluten.

- **Monitor nutrient intake** for potential deficiencies, especially for calcium, B12, and omega-3s.

- **Keep a food diary** to track your meals and any reactions or sensitivities that may arise.

Managing food allergies and sensitivities during pregnancy can be challenging, but with careful planning and a balanced, nutrient-rich diet, you can ensure both your health and the health of your baby. Being proactive and informed will help you navigate your pregnancy with confidence and peace of mind.

Vegan and Vegetarian Pregnancy Nutrition

Maintaining a vegan or vegetarian diet during pregnancy can be healthy and beneficial, but it requires careful planning to ensure that both you and your baby are receiving the necessary nutrients for proper development. Plant-based diets are rich in fiber, vitamins, and antioxidants, and they can help lower the risk of certain pregnancy-related complications, such as gestational diabetes and high blood pressure. However, due to the absence of animal-based products, you must pay extra attention to ensure you're getting enough protein, calcium, iron, vitamin B12, and omega-3 fatty acids.

The Importance of a Well-Balanced Vegan or Vegetarian Diet

During pregnancy, your body's nutritional needs are significantly increased, and it's crucial to meet these demands for both your health and the health of your baby. If you're following a vegan or vegetarian diet, you may be more prone to deficiencies in key nutrients, which can have implications for your pregnancy.

Protein is essential for fetal growth and development. It supports the formation of organs, muscles, and tissues. Plant-based proteins are often incomplete, meaning they don't contain all nine essential amino acids your body needs. To ensure adequate protein intake, you need to include a variety of protein sources in your diet, such as legumes, lentils, tofu, tempeh, quinoa, and seitan.

Calcium is necessary for the development of your baby's bones and teeth. Without enough calcium, your body will take calcium from your bones, which can weaken them. While dairy is a common source of calcium, there are plenty of plant-based sources available, including fortified plant milks and leafy greens.

Iron is vital for the production of hemoglobin, the protein in red blood cells that carries oxygen to your baby. Plant-based iron (non-heme iron) is not as easily absorbed as the iron found in animal products (heme iron), so you must consume higher amounts of plant-based iron sources, like spinach, lentils, beans, fortified cereals, and pumpkin seeds. Pairing these foods with a source of vitamin C, such as oranges or bell peppers, can help enhance iron absorption.

Vitamin B12 is one of the most crucial nutrients for pregnant women, as it supports brain function and the formation of red blood cells.

Omega-3 fatty acids, particularly DHA and EPA, play a significant role in brain development and can help reduce the risk of preterm birth. While omega-3s are commonly found in fatty fish, plant-based sources like flaxseeds and chia seeds can provide these essential fats.

Practical Tips for Meeting Nutritional Needs on a Plant-Based Diet

Meeting your nutritional needs on a vegan or vegetarian diet requires planning, but it is entirely achievable with the right strategies.

1. Incorporate Diverse Protein Sources

Protein is crucial during pregnancy to support both your baby's growth and your body's increased demands. Try combining different plant-based protein sources to ensure you're getting a complete amino acid profile. Some great protein-packed foods to include are:

- Legumes (beans, lentils, chickpeas)
- Tofu and tempeh
- Seitan (wheat protein)

2. Quinoa, edamame, and hemp seeds

Nut butters (almond butter, peanut butter) These foods can be incorporated into salads, soups, stir-fries, and wraps, or used as the main base for various dishes.

3. Ensure Sufficient Iron Intake

Iron is one nutrient where vegetarians and vegans often fall short, so it's crucial to focus on iron-rich plant foods. Here's how to boost your iron intake:

- Include iron-rich foods like lentils, beans, tofu, quinoa, and fortified cereals in your meals.
- Pair these with vitamin C-rich foods (like oranges, bell peppers, broccoli, or strawberries) to improve iron absorption.
- Avoid drinking coffee or tea with meals, as these beverages can inhibit iron absorption. Instead, drink water or herbal teas that don't contain tannins.

4. Get Enough Calcium and Vitamin D

Without dairy products, it's essential to find alternative sources of calcium. Look for fortified plant milks (such as almond, soy, or oat milk), leafy greens like kale and collard greens, and calcium-set tofu. Vitamin D is also necessary for calcium absorption, so ensure you get enough, including fortified foods (like fortified plant milks or cereals), mushrooms exposed to sunlight, or consider a vitamin D supplement based on your doctor's recommendation.

5. Supplement with Vitamin B12

Vitamin B12 is essential for the health of both you and your baby, but it is not naturally found in plant-based foods. You can obtain B12 through fortified foods such as nutritional yeast, fortified cereals, and fortified plant milks. In many cases, a B12 supplement is recommended for vegans, so discuss this with your healthcare provider to ensure you're getting enough.

6. Omega-3 Fatty Acids and DHA

Omega-3 fatty acids are crucial for your baby's brain and eye development. If you don't consume fish, it's important to include plant-based sources of omega-3s, such as flaxseeds, chia seeds, walnuts, and hemp seeds. You can also consider taking an algae-based DHA supplement, which is a plant-based source of the essential omega-3 fatty acids.

7. Stay Hydrated

A vegan or vegetarian diet often includes more fiber, which can be very beneficial for digestion but may also require increased water intake. Ensure you're drinking plenty of fluids to stay hydrated and support your body's increased blood volume during pregnancy.

Strategic Suggestions

- **Consult a healthcare provider or dietitian** to ensure your vegan or vegetarian diet is balanced and providing all the necessary nutrients for both you and your baby.
- **Diversify your protein sources,** including a variety of legumes, seeds, tofu, and grains to meet your amino acid needs.

- **Take a B12 supplement** and ensure you are consuming fortified foods like plant milks or nutritional yeast.
- **Pair iron-rich foods with vitamin C** to enhance iron absorption and avoid consuming iron-rich foods with coffee or tea.
- **Consider algae-based omega-3 supplements** to meet your DHA and EPA needs for brain development.
- **Drink plenty of water to stay hydrated**, especially if you're consuming higher amounts of fiber.

With careful planning, a vegan or vegetarian diet can absolutely support a healthy pregnancy. The key is making sure you're consuming a variety of nutrient-dense foods, staying mindful of your intake of essential vitamins and minerals, and working with a healthcare provider to ensure you're meeting all your nutritional needs.

Chapter 6: Foods to Avoid During Pregnancy

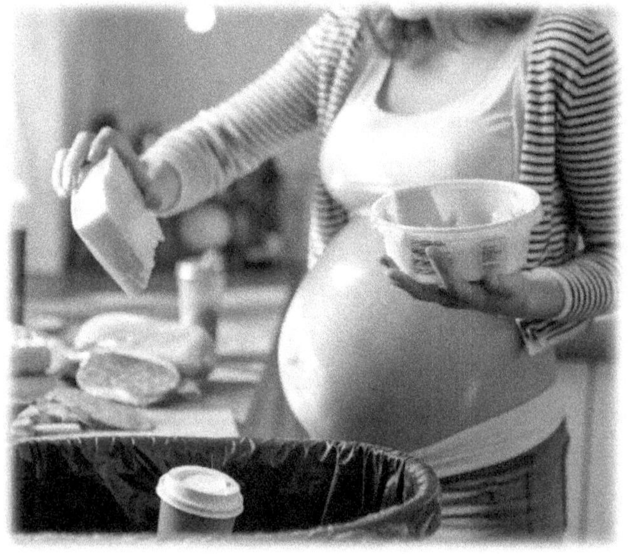

Pregnancy is a delicate time when both the mother and baby's health require careful attention. A balanced, nutritious diet supports a healthy pregnancy, but some foods pose risks to both. Identifying and avoiding these foods is essential to ensure the well-being of both mother and child throughout this critical period.

Harmful Foods and Ingredients: What to Steer Clear Of

Pregnancy is a time when you need to pay extra attention to what you eat. Certain foods and ingredients can pose risks to you and your baby's health, so it's essential to be aware of what to avoid. While you may already have a general idea of healthy eating, understanding which foods can be harmful during pregnancy is crucial for ensuring the well-being of both you and your developing baby. Below, we will explore some of the most important foods and ingredients to steer clear of while pregnant.

Foods to Avoid for a Healthy Pregnancy

1. Unpasteurized Dairy Products

Unpasteurized or raw dairy products—like milk, cheese, and yogurt—can be harmful during pregnancy because they may contain Listeria, a bacteria that can cause a serious infection known as listeriosis. This infection can lead to miscarriage, stillbirth, or severe illness in newborns. Common unpasteurized cheeses include Brie, Camembert, Roquefort, and some soft cheeses. Always choose pasteurized dairy products to lower the risk of listeriosis.

2. Raw or Undercooked Meat, Poultry, and Seafood

Consuming raw or undercooked meat, poultry, or seafood puts you at risk for foodborne illnesses, such as Salmonella, Toxoplasmosis, and Listeria, all of which can seriously harm both you and your baby. It's important to ensure that meat, poultry, and seafood are cooked thoroughly. For meat, this means no pink in the center and reaching the correct internal temperatures (e.g., 165°F for chicken).

3. Certain Fish High in Mercury

Some types of fish can contain high levels of mercury, which can negatively affect your baby's developing nervous system. Fish like shark, swordfish, king mackerel, and tilefish are known to have higher mercury content. Instead, opt for low-mercury fish such as salmon, shrimp, tilapia, and cod. Eating fish can still be healthy during pregnancy, but moderation is key to avoid excess mercury buildup.

4. Raw Eggs

Raw or undercooked eggs are another food to avoid due to the risk of Salmonella infection. Many homemade dishes, such as mayonnaise, hollandaise sauce, and some desserts like mousse, may contain raw eggs. To stay safe, use pasteurized eggs in recipes that call for raw eggs, or avoid these types of dishes altogether during your pregnancy.

5. Unwashed Fruits and Vegetables

While fruits and vegetables are essential to a healthy pregnancy, they need to be thoroughly washed before consumption. Unwashed produce can carry bacteria, pesticides, and parasites like Toxoplasma or Listeria, which may harm your pregnancy. Always wash your fruits and vegetables under running water, and if possible, peel or scrub them before eating.

6. Caffeine

While a small cup of coffee or tea may seem like a harmless treat, excessive caffeine intake during pregnancy can lead to complications. High caffeine levels can increase the risk of miscarriage, low birth weight, and preterm birth. It is advised to limit your caffeine intake to no more than 200 milligrams per day, which is about the amount in one 12-ounce cup of coffee. Keep in mind that caffeine is also found in chocolate, some sodas, and certain medications, so be mindful of your total daily intake.

7. Alcohol

Alcohol consumption during pregnancy can cause serious developmental issues in your baby, including fetal alcohol syndrome, which can lead to lifelong physical and mental disabilities. No amount of alcohol has been proven safe during pregnancy, so it's best to completely avoid alcohol while you are pregnant. Even small amounts of alcohol can have harmful effects on your baby, especially during the first trimester when major organs are developing.

8. Processed Junk Foods

Although they may be tempting, heavily processed foods are best avoided during pregnancy. These foods often contain unhealthy fats, high levels of sodium, sugar, and artificial ingredients, which can contribute to excessive weight gain, high blood pressure, and gestational diabetes. Opt for whole, nutrient-dense foods like fruits, vegetables, whole grains, and lean proteins.

9. Artificial Sweeteners

Some artificial sweeteners, such as aspartame and sucralose, have been linked to potential risks during pregnancy. While research on the safety of artificial sweeteners during pregnancy is ongoing, it's wise to limit their use. Instead, choose natural sweeteners like honey or stevia in moderation. Also, keep in mind that many sugar-free products still contain sugar alcohols like sorbitol, which can cause digestive issues like bloating and gas.

10. Canned Foods with BPA

Bisphenol A (BPA) is a chemical used in the lining of some food cans, and it can leach into food, particularly acidic foods like tomatoes. BPA has been associated with developmental and reproductive issues, so it's a good idea to limit your exposure. Opt for BPA-free cans or choose fresh, frozen, or glass-packed alternatives when possible.

Strategic Suggestions

- **Stick to pasteurized products:** Always choose pasteurized milk, cheese, and other dairy products to reduce the risk of foodborne illness.

- **Cook meat and seafood thoroughly:** Ensure that all meat and seafood are cooked to the proper internal temperatures to kill harmful bacteria and parasites.

- **Avoid high-mercury fish:** Choose low-mercury fish like salmon and shrimp to support your baby's development without risking mercury exposure.

- **Limit caffeine intake:** Keep your caffeine consumption under 200 milligrams per day, and be mindful of hidden sources like chocolate and some medications.

- **Avoid alcohol completely:** Do not consume any amount of alcohol during pregnancy to ensure your baby's safety and development.

- **Choose whole, natural foods:** Opt for fresh fruits, vegetables, and whole grains, and limit processed foods and artificial sweeteners.

- **Wash your produce thoroughly:** Always wash fruits and vegetables before eating to eliminate the risk of harmful bacteria or pesticides.

- **Consider BPA-free alternatives:** Choose BPA-free canned goods or opt for fresh, frozen, or glass-packaged foods to reduce exposure to harmful chemicals.

Being mindful of these foods and ingredients during pregnancy will help you ensure a safer, healthier experience for both you and your baby. A little extra care in the kitchen goes a long way in providing the nutrition and protection needed for a healthy pregnancy.

Understanding the Risks of Mercury and Contaminated Foods

Mercury contamination is a significant concern during pregnancy, especially when it comes to certain types of fish. Mercury is a toxic metal that can accumulate in your body over time, leading to potential risks for both you and your baby. It's important to understand which foods can carry higher levels of mercury and how to minimize exposure to ensure a healthy pregnancy.

What Is Mercury, and Why Is It Dangerous During Pregnancy?

Mercury is a naturally occurring element found in the environment. It exists in different forms, but the most concerning type for pregnant women is methylmercury. Methylmercury is found primarily in certain fish and seafood. When you eat contaminated fish, mercury can enter your bloodstream and pass through the placenta to your developing baby.

The risks of mercury exposure during pregnancy are significant because it can interfere with the development of your baby's brain and nervous system. High levels of mercury can lead to developmental delays, learning disabilities, and even damage to the baby's hearing and vision. The effects of mercury poisoning can be long-lasting and may impact cognitive function, motor skills, and behavior. That's why it's critical to be mindful of mercury exposure during pregnancy and take steps to minimize your intake.

Which Fish Contain the Most Mercury?

Certain types of fish are more likely to contain higher levels of mercury due to their size, age, and diet. Larger fish that are at the top of the food chain tend to accumulate more mercury. These include:

1. Shark

Shark is one of the fish most likely to contain high levels of mercury. Due to its large size and long lifespan, it absorbs a significant amount of mercury from the environment and its prey.

2. Swordfish

Swordfish is another fish known to have high mercury levels. Like shark, swordfish is a large, predatory fish that tends to accumulate mercury in its tissues.

3. King Mackerel

King mackerel is a large fish that also tends to contain elevated mercury levels. While mackerel is generally healthy, this particular variety should be avoided during pregnancy.

4. Tilefish

Tilefish, especially those found in the Gulf of Mexico, have been found to contain dangerous levels of mercury. It's best to avoid this type of fish during pregnancy.

5. Albacore Tuna (canned)

While tuna is a popular fish, it is essential to limit your intake of albacore tuna, which contains more mercury than light tuna. Canned albacore tuna, in particular, can be a significant source of mercury.

What About Low-Mercury Fish?

While high-mercury fish should be avoided, there are plenty of fish that are safe and even beneficial for you and your baby. Many types of fish are rich in omega-3 fatty acids, which are important for your baby's brain and eye development. The key is to choose fish with lower mercury levels. These include:

1. Salmon

Salmon is one of the most well-known and highly recommended sources of omega-3 fatty acids, particularly DHA (docosahexaenoic acid) and EPA (eicosapentaenoic acid), which are the two most bioavailable forms of omega-3s for human health. It is a great choice for your pregnancy diet.

2. Shrimp

Shrimp is another safe seafood option with little to no mercury. It's low in fat and high in protein, making it a healthy choice.

3. Tilapia

Tilapia is low in mercury and a good source of lean protein. It's a versatile fish that can be used in various recipes.

4. Cod

Cod is a mild-tasting fish that is low in mercury and provides a good amount of protein. It can be easily incorporated into your meals.

5. Sardines

Sardines are small fish that have a low mercury content and are packed with omega-3 fatty acids, vitamin D, and calcium. They're a great addition to your pregnancy diet.

6. Anchovie

Like sardines, anchovies are small fish that have minimal mercury exposure. They are rich in omega-3s and can be used in salads, pasta dishes, or on pizzas.

How to Minimize Mercury Exposure

While fish and seafood can be part of a healthy pregnancy diet, it's important to take steps to limit your mercury exposure. Here are some practical tips to help you reduce your risks:

1. Limit High-Mercury Fish

As mentioned earlier, avoid fish like shark, swordfish, king mackerel, and tilefish. These fish contain the highest levels of mercury, so it's best to exclude them entirely from your diet during pregnancy.

2. Choose Low-Mercury Fish

Opt for fish that are lower in mercury, such as salmon, shrimp, tilapia, and cod. These fish are rich in essential nutrients like omega-3 fatty acids and protein while keeping mercury exposure to a minimum.

3. Check Local Fish Advisories

If you live near a body of water and like to catch your own fish, it's important to check local fish advisories. Some lakes, rivers, and coastal areas may have higher mercury levels in certain fish species, so always be informed about the safety of consuming locally caught fish.

4. Limit Tuna Consumption

Tuna is a popular fish, but it's important to limit your intake of albacore (white) tuna, which contains more mercury than light tuna. If you enjoy canned tuna, try to stick to the light variety and keep your consumption to no more than 2-3 servings per week.

5. Opt for Organic or Wild-Caught Fish

When possible, choose wild-caught fish over farmed fish. Wild-caught fish are less likely to have been exposed to environmental pollutants, including mercury. Additionally, consider organic or sustainably farmed fish options, as these may have fewer contaminants.

6. Diversify Your Protein Sources

While fish is a great source of protein, it's important to diversify your protein intake to avoid overconsumption of any one type of food. Other protein sources include beans, nuts, seeds, eggs, and lean meats.

7. Keep Portion Sizes in Mind

Moderation is key when it comes to fish consumption. Even when choosing low-mercury fish, keep your portions to a reasonable size. The FDA recommends 2-3 servings (8-12 ounces) of low-mercury fish per week during pregnancy.

Strategic Suggestions

- **Stick to fish with low mercury content**, like salmon, tilapia, and shrimp.
- **Avoid high-mercury fish** such as shark, swordfish, and tilefish.
- **Limit albacore tuna** to one serving a week and opt for light tuna.
- **Diversify your protein sources** to reduce the risk of mercury exposure.
- **Always check local fish advisories** if you catch your own fish.
- **Choose wild-caught or sustainably farmed fish** when possible.

Being aware of mercury risks and making informed choices about the fish you eat during pregnancy is crucial for the health of both you and your baby. Follow these guidelines to safely enjoy the benefits of fish while minimizing your exposure to harmful mercury.

Caffeine and Alcohol: Setting Healthy Limits

During pregnancy, you may be wondering about the safety of consuming caffeine and alcohol. These substances are commonly consumed in various forms, such as coffee, tea, soda, and alcoholic beverages. However, it's essential to understand the impact they can have on your health and your baby's development. While occasional, moderate consumption might be acceptable for some pregnant women, it's important to be mindful of your intake and set healthy limits.

Caffeine During Pregnancy: Is It Safe?

Caffeine is a stimulant found in coffee, tea, chocolate, soda, and even some medications. It can cross the placenta and reach your baby, which is a concern since your baby's developing organs, including their brain, may not be equipped to metabolize caffeine efficiently. Although small amounts of caffeine are generally considered safe during pregnancy, consuming too much can lead to potential risks.

One of the primary concerns regarding caffeine intake during pregnancy is its effect on the developing fetus. High caffeine consumption has been linked to an increased risk of miscarriage, low birth weight, preterm birth, and developmental delays. Additionally, excessive caffeine intake can contribute to dehydration, which can lead to complications like preterm labor or an increased risk of urinary tract infections.

How Much Caffeine Is Safe?

Health experts, including the American College of Obstetricians and Gynecologists (ACOG), recommend limiting caffeine intake to no more than 200 milligrams per day during pregnancy. This is roughly the amount in one 12-ounce cup of coffee, though it can vary depending on the type of coffee or tea. Keep in mind that caffeine is present in many foods and beverages, not just coffee. For example:

- A 12-ounce can of cola typically contains around 30-40 milligrams of caffeine.

- A 16-ounce serving of iced tea can have anywhere from 40-70 milligrams of caffeine.

- A cup of hot chocolate may contain 5-20 milligrams, depending on the type.

Energy drinks and some medications can contain significant amounts of caffeine, so always check labels carefully.

Caffeine and Your Baby's Development

Although caffeine is a natural substance, your baby's developing nervous system is particularly sensitive to it. The ability to metabolize caffeine doesn't fully develop until later in pregnancy, so excessive amounts can have a greater impact earlier on. Research has shown that high caffeine intake during pregnancy can result in the following:

1. Increased Risk of Miscarriage

Studies have shown that consuming more than 200 milligrams of caffeine daily can increase the risk of miscarriage, especially during the first trimester when your baby's organs are developing.

2. Low Birth Weight

Babies born to mothers who consume high amounts of caffeine during pregnancy may be born with low birth weight, which can lead to complications, such as difficulty maintaining body temperature, feeding problems, and an increased risk of infections.

3. Premature Birth

Excessive caffeine intake has been linked to a slightly increased risk of preterm birth. It's important to remember that preterm birth can lead to a variety of health concerns for your baby, including underdeveloped lungs and other vital organs.

4. Developmental Delays

High caffeine consumption may impact your baby's brain development. Some studies suggest that children exposed to high caffeine levels in utero may experience developmental delays or behavioral issues later in life.

Alcohol During Pregnancy: The Risks and Limits

Alcohol is another substance that should be avoided during pregnancy due to its potential to cause harm to your baby. When you drink alcohol, it passes through the placenta and reaches your baby, whose liver is not yet developed enough to process it. Even small amounts of alcohol during pregnancy can be harmful to your baby and pose serious risks to their development. While some may think occasional or light drinking is safe, no amount of alcohol has been proven to be completely safe during pregnancy.

Drinking alcohol during pregnancy can cause:

1. Fetal Alcohol Spectrum Disorders (FASDs)

The most severe consequence of alcohol consumption during pregnancy is Fetal Alcohol Syndrome (FAS). This condition can cause a range of physical, behavioral, and intellectual disabilities in children, including facial abnormalities, developmental delays, learning difficulties, and attention problems.

2. Miscarriage and Stillbirth

Alcohol consumption increases the risk of miscarriage and stillbirth, particularly in the early stages of pregnancy when your baby's vital organs are developing.

3. Premature Birth and Low Birth Weight

Drinking alcohol during pregnancy can also increase the likelihood of premature birth and low birth weight, which can lead to complications for your baby after birth.

4. Neurological Impairment

Alcohol can severely interfere with your baby's brain development during pregnancy, leading to a range of long-term cognitive and developmental issues that can affect the child for their entire life.

Setting Healthy Limits for Caffeine and Alcohol

To ensure the best outcome for both you and your baby, it's crucial to make informed decisions about caffeine and alcohol consumption during pregnancy. Here are some strategies to help you set healthy limits:

1. Monitor Your Caffeine Intake

If you're a coffee or tea drinker, keep track of your daily intake and make sure you don't exceed 200 milligrams of caffeine. Consider switching to decaffeinated beverages or herbal teas, which can be just as satisfying without the caffeine. Be mindful of hidden sources of caffeine, such as sodas, energy drinks, and even some over-the-counter medications.

2. Opt for Caffeine-Free Alternatives

There are plenty of caffeine-free alternatives that can help you stay hydrated and feel refreshed during pregnancy. Try flavored water, fruit-infused water, or caffeine-free herbal teas like peppermint or ginger, which can also help with nausea or digestion.

3. Avoid Alcohol Completely

The safest choice during pregnancy is to avoid alcohol entirely. There's no known safe amount of alcohol during pregnancy, and even small amounts can have an impact on your baby's health.

4. Communicate with Your Healthcare Provider

If you have concerns about caffeine or alcohol consumption, discuss them with your healthcare provider. They can offer personalized advice and help you set realistic, safe limits based on your specific situation.

Strategic Suggestions

- **Limit caffeine intake** to no more than 200 milligrams per day (about one cup of coffee).

- **Avoid alcohol completely** during pregnancy to prevent any risks to your baby.

- **Stay hydrated with caffeine-free alternatives** like herbal teas, flavored water, or fresh fruit juices.

- **Check labels for hidden sources of caffeine**, especially in sodas, energy drinks, and medications.

If you struggle with reducing caffeine, consider gradually cutting back to prevent withdrawal symptoms like headaches or fatigue.

Reach out to your healthcare provider if you have concerns about your caffeine or alcohol consumption during pregnancy.

Manage your caffeine and alcohol intake carefully to reduce the risks to both you and your baby. Focusing on healthy hydration options and making mindful choices will ensure a safer and more enjoyable pregnancy experience.

Chapter 7: Common Pregnancy Cravings and Healthy Substitutions

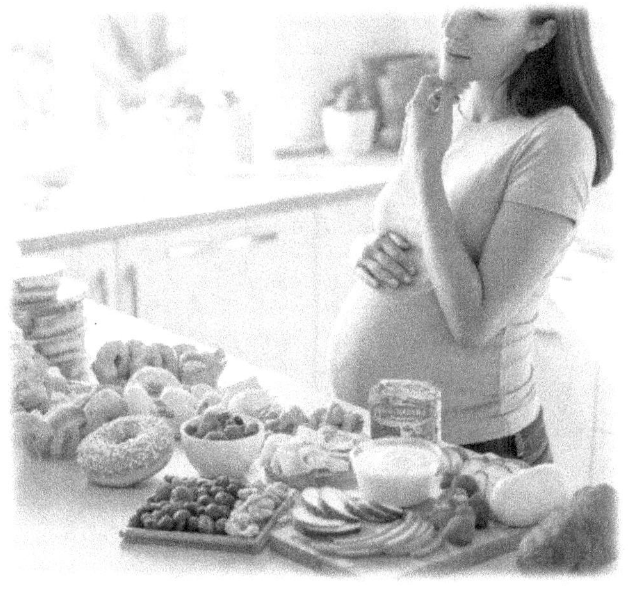

Weight management during pregnancy involves gaining the right amount of weight to support your baby's growth and your health. It's essential to balance proper nutrition and physical activity to ensure a healthy pregnancy while avoiding excessive weight gain or undernutrition. Healthy weight management contributes to a positive pregnancy outcome.

Understanding the Science Behind Pregnancy Cravings

Pregnancy cravings are a well-known phenomenon that many expecting mothers experience. These cravings can range from a sudden desire for sweet, salty, or unusual foods to even non-food items, known as pica. While cravings are often seen as an odd part of pregnancy, there is a scientific explanation for them. Understanding the causes behind these cravings can help you navigate them in a healthy way, ensuring both you and your baby receive the nutrition you need.

During pregnancy, your body undergoes a multitude of changes that affect your hormones, senses, and nutritional needs. One of the major contributors to cravings is the increase in hormones, particularly estrogen and progesterone, which are responsible for regulating your pregnancy. These hormones not only help in the development of the baby but also influence your appetite, food preferences, and taste.

Some researchers believe that cravings may be your body's way of signaling nutritional deficiencies. For instance, if you're craving citrus fruits, your body may be telling you that it needs more vitamin C. Similarly, cravings for salty foods could indicate a need for more sodium, which plays a role in maintaining fluid balance and blood pressure. However, it's important to note that cravings don't always directly correlate with nutritional needs. Many cravings are simply a response to changes in taste perception or emotional factors, such as stress or anxiety.

Another reason for cravings could be the heightened sense of smell and taste that often occurs during pregnancy. Many women report becoming more sensitive to certain smells and flavors, sometimes making previously loved foods unappealing while other, more unusual combinations seem irresistible. This could be your body's way of adjusting to changes in how food is perceived, possibly influencing your desire to try new or more intense flavors.

Stress is another contributor to pregnancy cravings. Pregnancy can be an emotional rollercoaster, and stress can trigger cravings for comfort foods, often those high in sugar, fat, or salt. This is because these foods activate the brain's reward system, releasing dopamine, a "feel-good" hormone. As a result, comfort foods become a quick way to relieve stress or anxiety, even though they might not be the best choice for your health or your baby's development.

The physical changes in your body can also cause cravings. The growing baby places pressure on your digestive system, which can affect your ability to digest certain foods. This might cause some women to crave foods that are easier to digest or foods that relieve nausea or indigestion, such as bland crackers or ginger. Hormonal shifts may also lead to changes in your blood sugar levels, influencing cravings for sugary or carb-rich foods to boost your energy.

In some cases, cravings can be linked to emotional changes. Pregnancy can be a time of heightened emotions, and many women crave certain foods as a form of comfort or to soothe anxiety. For instance, cravings for chocolate or ice cream may be your body's way of seeking an emotional boost. These cravings are often psychological rather than nutritional but can still be valid experiences.

While cravings are a normal part of pregnancy, they don't always need to be indulged in excess. It's essential to listen to your body but also to ensure that the foods you crave contribute positively to your health and your baby's development. Moderation is key.

Managing Cravings in a Healthy Way

Here are a few tips to manage cravings in a way that benefits both you and your baby:

1. Stay Hydrated

Sometimes, what feels like a craving might simply be thirst. Ensure that you're drinking enough water throughout the day to help reduce unnecessary cravings.

2. Balanced Meals

Eat nutrient-dense meals that include a balance of protein, healthy fats, and complex carbohydrates. This can help stabilize blood sugar levels and reduce the intensity of cravings.

3. Healthy Substitutes

If you're craving something sweet, consider healthier alternatives like fresh fruit, yogurt with honey, or smoothies made with fruits and greens. If you're craving salty foods, try whole-grain crackers or nuts instead of chips.

4. Mindful Eating

Practice mindful eating to truly savor your food. This can help you recognize when you're eating out of hunger versus when you're eating due to a craving, helping you avoid overeating.

5. Don't Deny Yourself

If the craving is strong, allow yourself a small portion of the food you're craving. Completely denying yourself may lead to feelings of deprivation, which could cause you to overindulge later. Moderation is the key.

Conclusion

Understanding the science behind pregnancy cravings helps you recognize them as a natural part of the process. Make mindful choices and listening to your body to manage cravings while supporting both your nutritional needs and your baby's growth.

Strategic Suggestions

- **Keep Healthy Snacks Handy:** Stock your kitchen with healthier alternatives to curb cravings before they get overwhelming. This can include cut vegetables, nuts, seeds, or fruits.

- **Track Your Cravings:** Keep a journal of your cravings to identify any patterns. If you notice a regular craving for a particular food, try to figure out if it's linked to a specific nutrient or emotional need.

- **Eat Smaller, Frequent Meals:** This helps keep blood sugar levels stable, preventing extreme hunger and the subsequent onset of strong cravings.

- **Exercise:** Gentle exercise, like walking or yoga, can help release endorphins, reducing stress and helping to prevent emotional cravings.

Healthy Alternatives to Sugar and Processed Foods

During pregnancy, you might find yourself craving sweet, sugary, or processed foods, but indulging in these too frequently can have negative effects on both your health and your baby's development. Excess sugar and processed foods are not only empty in terms of nutrition, but they can also contribute to weight gain, increased blood sugar levels, and other complications. Thankfully, there are many healthy alternatives to satisfy those cravings while still giving your body the nutrients it needs to thrive during this important time.

The Risks of Excess Sugar and Processed Foods

Excessive sugar intake during pregnancy can lead to various complications, including gestational diabetes, high blood pressure, and increased risk of preterm labor. Processed foods, which are often high in sodium, unhealthy fats, and refined sugars, can also contribute to inflammation, digestive problems, and poor fetal development. Moreover, consuming too much sugar can spike your blood glucose levels, which not only affects your energy levels but can also put unnecessary strain on your insulin system.

Processed foods, such as packaged snacks, cookies, chips, and sugary drinks, often lack essential nutrients like fiber, vitamins, and minerals. When you're eating these foods, you're essentially filling your body with "empty" calories that offer little to no nutritional value. This is especially concerning during pregnancy when both you and your baby require extra nourishment for optimal health and growth.

The good news is, there are numerous healthier, more nutrient-rich alternatives that can help you curb cravings for sugary and processed foods. These options are rich in vitamins, minerals, fiber, and healthy fats, which will help ensure you're getting the right nutrients, not just empty calories.

Healthy Substitutes for Sugar and Processed Foods

1. Fresh Fruits for Sweet Cravings

When you're craving something sweet, reach for a piece of fresh fruit instead of processed sweets like candy or sugary desserts. Fruits like berries, apples, and citrus are packed with vitamins and antioxidants that are beneficial for both you and your baby. They provide natural sugars that won't spike your blood sugar levels as rapidly as refined sugars and are high in fiber, which helps maintain good digestion. Fresh fruit is also a great source of vitamin C, which supports a healthy immune system.

For example, if you're craving something like chocolate, consider making a smoothie with frozen bananas, berries, and a tablespoon of cocoa powder. The natural sweetness of the fruit, combined with the rich flavor of cocoa, can satisfy your chocolate craving without all the extra sugar and unhealthy fats.

2. Yogurt as a Substitute for Processed Snacks

Instead of reaching for sugary snack bars or candy, try a bowl of plain Greek yogurt with fresh fruit, a drizzle of honey, or some unsweetened granola. Greek yogurt is a great source of protein, calcium, and probiotics, which are important for both your bone health and your gut. Ass fresh fruit or a small amount of honey to get a sweet treat without all the refined sugars found in processed snacks.

Opt for full-fat or low-fat Greek yogurt, depending on your nutritional needs. This helps promote better digestion and provides healthy fats that are essential for your body during pregnancy.

3. Homemade Energy Bites or Bars

Instead of buying processed granola bars, make your own energy bites using ingredients like oats, nut butter, honey, and chia seeds. These homemade treats are packed with healthy fats, fiber, and protein, making them a nutritious snack to keep your energy levels stable throughout the day. Plus, when you make them at home, you control what goes into them, ensuring there are no added sugars or preservatives.

4. Nuts and Seeds for Salty Cravings

If you're craving something salty, choose nuts and seeds like almonds, walnuts, or sunflower seeds. These are not only nutrient-dense but also provide healthy fats that are important for your baby's brain development.

5. Vegetable Chips Instead of Potato Chips

If you're craving something crunchy, consider making your own vegetable chips at home. You can bake thin slices of sweet potatoes, kale, or zucchini with a small amount of olive oil and seasoning. These homemade veggie chips are high in fiber, vitamins, and minerals while being much healthier than traditional potato chips, which are high in unhealthy fats and sodium.

6. Dark Chocolate for a Sweet Treat

When your craving for chocolate hits, choose dark chocolate over milk chocolate or sugary candy bars. Dark chocolate contains antioxidants and is lower in sugar, making it a healthier choice for satisfying that sweet tooth. Opt for chocolate that contains at least 70% cocoa, as this will have less sugar and more health benefits. A couple of squares of dark chocolate can be just enough to curb your cravings.

The Importance of Moderation

While it's perfectly normal to crave sweet or salty foods during pregnancy, it's essential to balance these cravings with nutritious options.

Moderation is key. It's okay to indulge in your cravings occasionally, but try to make healthier choices the majority of the time to ensure you're giving your body the best possible nutrition.

Initiate simple substitutions like choosing fresh fruits, homemade snacks, and nutrient-dense options to satisfy your cravings while promoting better health for yourself and your baby. The goal is to enjoy what you eat without compromising your nutritional needs.

Strategic Suggestions

- **Keep Healthy Snacks Available:** Stock your kitchen with fresh fruits, nuts, and homemade energy bites to curb cravings without reaching for processed snacks.

- **Read Labels Carefully:** If you do choose packaged snacks, always check the ingredients list. Look for options that are lower in sugar and free from artificial additives.

- **Practice Portion Control:** When indulging in treats like dark chocolate, keep portion sizes small. A little bit can go a long way in satisfying cravings.
- **Stay Active:** Physical activity helps reduce cravings, improve mood, and maintain a healthy weight during pregnancy.

Make these simple changes to manage your cravings in a healthier way, ensuring that you and your baby receive the nutrients you both need for optimal health.

Satisfying Nutrient-Rich Cravings

During pregnancy, cravings for specific foods are common, and they can vary from a sudden desire for salty snacks to sweet treats. However, the key to a healthy pregnancy is to balance these cravings with nutrient-rich options. The body needs essential vitamins, minerals, and macronutrients to support both the growing baby and the mother's well-being. Knowing how to satisfy cravings in a way that nourishes you both is crucial.

Understanding Nutrient-Rich Cravings

Cravings during pregnancy are largely due to the body's need for specific nutrients. For example, you might crave foods high in calcium or iron when your body needs more of these nutrients. These cravings can also be triggered by hormonal fluctuations that occur as your pregnancy progresses, making certain foods more appealing.

While cravings are completely normal, it's important to choose healthier, nutrient-dense options to meet your nutritional needs. This ensures that you're not only satisfying your desire for a specific taste or texture but also feeding your body with the vitamins, minerals, and other nutrients necessary for your health and the baby's development.

Instead of giving in to unhealthy choices like chips, cookies, or candy, consider substituting them with foods that provide the same satisfaction but offer valuable nutrients.

Healthy Alternatives for Common Pregnancy Cravings

1. Sweet Cravings

It's common to crave something sweet, such as chocolate, ice cream, or pastries. Instead of reaching for processed sugary snacks, opt for nutrient-dense alternatives that can satisfy your sweet tooth while providing vitamins and minerals.

- **Fresh fruit:** Fruits like berries, apples, and pears are naturally sweet and high in fiber, which helps with digestion and keeps you feeling full longer. You can also try frozen fruit.

- **Greek yogurt with honey:** If you're craving something creamy and sweet, plain Greek yogurt is an excellent option. It's rich in protein and calcium, and you can add a drizzle of honey or top it with fresh fruit for added sweetness.

- **Homemade fruit smoothies:** Blend up some frozen fruits like bananas, berries, and mangoes with a bit of almond milk or yogurt for a nutrient-packed, naturally sweet treat.

2. Salty Cravings

Salt cravings can often indicate a need for more electrolytes or hydration, so it's important to find alternatives that offer both salty flavors and the nutrients your body needs.

- **Nuts and seeds:** Almonds, walnuts, and sunflower seeds are great sources of healthy fats, fiber, and protein. Choose unsalted versions to avoid excess sodium. You can also make your own homemade trail mix with dried fruit and a variety of nuts.

- **Vegetable chips:** If you're craving something crunchy, baked vegetable chips made from sweet potatoes, zucchini, or kale can be a healthier substitute for regular chips. These options are high in fiber and antioxidants while providing that satisfying salty crunch.

- **Hummus and veggies:** A great way to satisfy a salty craving while getting in some veggies is to dip raw carrot sticks, cucumbers, or bell peppers in hummus. The healthy fats in the hummus and the fiber in the vegetables make this snack a great nutrient-rich option.

3. Crunchy Cravings

Pregnant women often crave something crunchy. This can be your body's way of needing a texture that offers a bit of a chew without being overly sweet or heavy.

- **Popcorn:** Air-popped popcorn is a fantastic low-calorie option that gives you that crunchy texture you might be craving. It's high in fiber and can be seasoned with a bit of olive oil and nutritional yeast for a savory, nutrient-dense snack.

- **Apple slices with almond butter:** Slicing up an apple and pairing it with a spoonful of almond butter offers a crunchy yet satisfying snack that also provides healthy fats and fiber. The combination of natural sweetness and crunch can hit the spot without overindulging in processed snacks.

4. Chocolate Cravings

Chocolate cravings are common during pregnancy, often because of hormonal changes, but indulging in sugary, processed chocolate bars isn't the best choice for you or your baby.

- **Dark chocolate:** Opt for dark chocolate with at least 70% cocoa. Dark chocolate is lower in sugar and offers antioxidants that help combat free radicals in your body. Just a small square can curb that craving without going overboard on sugar.

- **Homemade chocolate avocado mousse:** For a creamy, indulgent treat that's nutrient-rich, try making chocolate mousse with avocado, cocoa powder, and a touch of honey. Avocados provide healthy fats, while the cocoa satisfies your chocolate craving.

5. Carb Cravings

Carbohydrate cravings, such as for pasta, bread, or rice, are another common desire during pregnancy. Instead of opting for refined carbs, opt for whole grains or nutrient-dense options.

- **Sweet potato:** Sweet potatoes are high in fiber and vitamin A. They also offer a natural sweetness, which makes them a great alternative to traditional white potatoes or carb-heavy snacks.
- **Quinoa or brown rice:** Whole grains like quinoa and brown rice provide more fiber, protein, and essential minerals than refined grains. Quinoa is also a complete protein, making it especially beneficial during pregnancy.

Tips for Managing Cravings in a Nutrient-Rich Way

- **Stay Hydrated**

Sometimes cravings, especially for salty or sweet foods, causes dehydration. Make sure to drink plenty of water throughout the day. Aim for at least 8–10 glasses of water daily.

- **Eat Regular, Balanced Meals**

Skipping meals can make cravings worse. Eating smaller, balanced meals throughout the day helps keep your blood sugar levels stable and prevents excessive cravings.

- **Savor Your Cravings in Moderation**

If you really want a treat, allow yourself to enjoy it in moderation. Cravings are normal, but limiting the frequency of indulgent choices helps ensure that you stay on track with a balanced, nutritious diet.

- **Plan Ahead**

Keeping healthy snacks readily available is an effective strategy to help curb cravings before they become too intense. It's easy to reach for unhealthy options when hunger strikes, but having nutritious snacks on hand can prevent you from making impulsive, less beneficial choices. Having fruit, nuts, or homemade energy bites on hand can help you make better food choices when cravings strike.

Strategic Suggestions

- **Choose Nutrient-Dense Foods:** Opt for foods that satisfy cravings while also providing essential nutrients, such as fiber, healthy fats, and vitamins.

- **Practice Portion Control:** Enjoy treats in moderation. A small serving of dark chocolate or a handful of nuts can be more than enough to curb your craving.

- **Stay Hydrated:** Drinking plenty of water can help reduce the intensity of cravings, especially for salty or sweet foods.

- **Make Substitutions:** For every craving, think of a healthier substitute. Swap processed snacks for whole, fresh alternatives like fruits, veggies, and nuts.

Balancing cravings with healthy alternatives ensures that both you and your baby get the nourishment needed for optimal health and development during pregnancy.

Chapter 8: Weight Management During Pregnancy

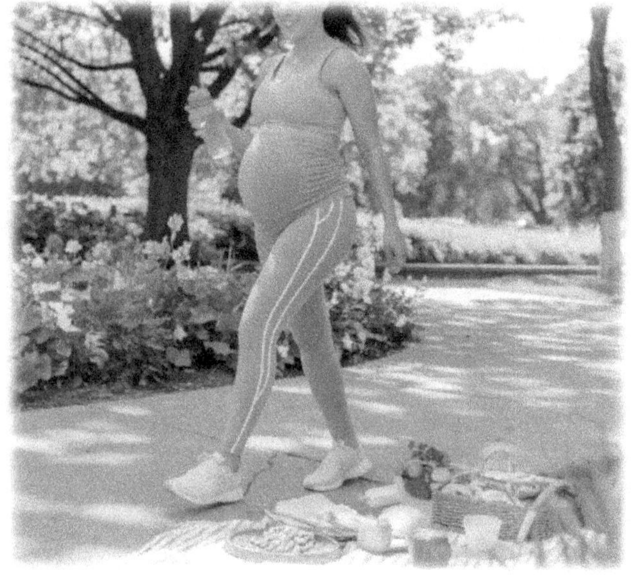

Weight management during pregnancy involves gaining the right amount of weight to support your baby's growth and your health. It's essential to balance proper nutrition and physical activity to ensure a healthy pregnancy while avoiding excessive weight gain or undernutrition. Healthy weight management contributes to a positive pregnancy outcome.

Healthy Weight Gain Guidelines for Each Trimester

Pregnancy is a time of change, and one of the most noticeable changes is weight gain. It's important to gain weight gradually and healthily to ensure both your well-being and the health of your baby. Every pregnancy is unique, but understanding the recommended weight gain guidelines for each trimester can help you manage your expectations and support a healthy pregnancy. Weight gain during pregnancy is not just about numbers; it's about supporting the development of your baby and preparing your body for childbirth.

Understanding Healthy Weight Gain During Pregnancy

When you're pregnant, your body undergoes many changes to nourish your growing baby. You may wonder how much weight gain is considered healthy and normal. The amount of weight you should gain depends on several factors, including your starting weight, your body's unique needs, and your health conditions.

In general, for a woman with a healthy pre-pregnancy weight (BMI between 18.5 and 24.9), the recommended weight gain is typically between 25 and 35 pounds during the course of the pregnancy. However, if you're underweight, you might need to gain more, and if you're overweight, you may need to gain less. If you have multiples (twins or more), your weight gain may need to be higher as well.

During the first trimester, you may not notice significant weight changes, and that's okay. Early on, the baby is still very small and doesn't require too many extra calories. Many women also experience morning sickness during this time, which can make eating more difficult. As a result, weight gain in the first trimester may be minimal or even slightly negative for some. By the second trimester, however, your appetite may increase, and your baby will begin growing faster, requiring more calories and nutrients.

Weight Gain Guidelines for Each Trimester

First Trimester (Weeks 1-12):

In the first trimester, most women gain only a small amount of weight—typically between 1 to 4 pounds. While it may feel like a lot, the initial weight gain often comes from increased blood volume, the growth of the placenta, and your body's adjustments to pregnancy hormones. It's important to focus on eating nutrient-dense foods that will support your baby's early development, even though you may not feel like eating much.

A healthy diet rich in folate (found in leafy greens, legumes, and fortified cereals), iron, and protein is essential during this stage. You don't need to increase your caloric intake significantly just yet, but small meals and snacks throughout the day can help meet your nutritional needs and keep you energized.

Second Trimester (Weeks 13-26):

During the second trimester, your baby grows rapidly, and you may notice an increase in your weight gain. Most women will gain between 1 to 2 pounds per week during this time. Expect to have gained about 12 to 14 pounds by the end of the second trimester.

This is a crucial period for your baby's growth, especially for the development of bones, muscles, and organs. It's important to get enough calcium and vitamin D, along with protein, to support these developments. At this stage, you may need around 300 extra calories per day, but focus on getting those extra calories from healthy sources like whole grains, lean proteins, fruits, and vegetables rather than sugary or fatty foods.

While it's normal to experience an increase in appetite, it's essential to listen to your body's cues. Aim for nutrient-dense meals to ensure that you're nourishing both yourself and your baby.

Third Trimester (Weeks 27-40):

The final trimester brings the most significant weight gain. You may gain about 1 pound per week, which could add up to about 10 to 15 pounds. At the end of your pregnancy, your baby would have grown large enough that most of the weight gain comes from the baby itself, along with increased amniotic fluid, breast tissue, and fat stores that prepare your body for breastfeeding.

Even though the weight gain is higher, it's important to continue focusing on a balanced diet. Your body needs plenty of energy and nutrients to support the baby's final growth phase and to prepare for labor. During this time, iron, calcium, and protein are especially important to maintain your energy levels and support fetal development.

You may feel full more quickly as your baby takes up more space in your abdomen, so try eating smaller meals more frequently. Hydration is also key during this trimester, as it helps with circulation, digestion, and the reduction of swelling, which is common during the final weeks of pregnancy.

Factors That Influence Weight Gain

Keep in mind that everyone's pregnancy is different. Genetics, lifestyle, and overall health will influence your weight gain. It's important not to compare yourself to others, as each woman's body responds to pregnancy differently. Some women may gain more weight than recommended, while others may gain less, and that's okay.

Conditions like gestational diabetes, high blood pressure, or carrying multiples can also affect how much weight you should gain, so always consult your doctor or midwife about your individual needs. They can guide you on how to adjust your diet and lifestyle to support a healthy pregnancy and ensure the best outcomes for both you and your baby.

Conclusion

In pregnancy, gaining the right amount of weight is important for both your health and your baby's development. Aim for steady weight gain, focusing on nutrient-rich foods and following the general guidelines for each trimester. With careful planning and attention to your body's needs, you can ensure that your weight gain supports a healthy pregnancy and sets you up for a positive postpartum experience.

Strategic Suggestions

- **Focus on whole, nutrient-dense foods**. Fruits, vegetables, lean proteins, whole grains, and healthy fats should make up most of your meals and snacks.
- **Stay hydrated, drinking plenty of water**, which can also help with common pregnancy symptoms like swelling and constipation.
- **Avoid excessive snacking** on sugary or highly processed foods. Instead,

choose healthy snacks like nuts, yogurt, or sliced veggies.

- **Listen to your body's hunger and fullness cues**. Eating slowly and eating smaller meals more often can help prevent overeating.

- **Keep track of your weight gain**, but don't obsess over the numbers. Trust your healthcare provider to guide you in the right direction.

Balancing Nutrient Intake with Calorie Needs

Maintaining a healthy pregnancy requires more than just eating for two. It's not only about how much you eat, but also about making sure you're consuming the right nutrients to support both your own health and your baby's growth. During pregnancy, your body's nutritional needs change, and it's important to balance your calorie intake with the right nutrients to ensure you're nourishing yourself and your baby.

Understanding Your Calorie Needs

Calories are units of energy that your body uses to perform daily functions. During pregnancy, your body requires additional energy to support your growing baby, but this doesn't mean you need to eat significantly more food. The amount of additional calories needed varies based on your individual needs and the stage of your pregnancy. Generally, you'll need about 300 extra calories per day in the second trimester and about 450 extra calories per day in the third trimester.

However, this doesn't mean you should simply eat more food indiscriminately. The key is to make these extra calories count. You want to consume nutrient-rich foods that provide essential vitamins, minerals, and healthy fats, rather than simply focusing on calories. This is where the concept of balancing nutrient intake becomes crucial.

Balancing Nutrients for Optimal Health

Pregnancy is a critical time for fetal development, and ensuring that your body gets the right combination of nutrients can positively impact both your health and the health of your baby. Here are the most important nutrients to focus on during pregnancy:

1. Protein

Protein is essential for your baby's growth, especially during the second and third trimesters. It's a building block for cells and tissues, and it helps develop your baby's muscles, organs, and immune system. You'll need about 70 to 100 grams of protein per day during pregnancy, depending on your weight and activity level. Excellent sources of protein include lean meats, eggs, dairy products, legumes, and tofu.

2. Calcium

Calcium is necessary for developing your baby's bones and teeth. It also plays a role in muscle function and nerve signaling. During pregnancy, you need about 1,000 milligrams of calcium per day, which can be met through dairy products like milk and yogurt, fortified plant-based milks, leafy green vegetables, almonds, and tofu.

3. Iron

Iron helps carry oxygen to your baby and prevents iron-deficiency anemia, which is common during pregnancy. Your body's blood volume increases, requiring more iron to maintain healthy circulation. Aim for around 27 milligrams of iron per day, which can be found in lean meats, beans, fortified cereals, spinach, and other green leafy vegetables.

4. Folate (Vitamin B9)

Folate is crucial for preventing birth defects, especially in the brain and spine. It helps in the production of red blood cells and the development of the neural tube. You should aim for 600 to 800 micrograms of folate each day, which can be found in leafy green vegetables, citrus fruits, beans, and fortified grains.

5. Healthy Fats

Your body needs fats for energy, but also for the proper functioning of cells and for the development of your baby's brain and nervous system. Healthy fats, like omega-3 fatty acids, are especially important for brain development. Foods rich in healthy fats include avocados, nuts, seeds, and fatty fish like salmon (which is also a great source of protein and calcium).

6. Vitamin D

Vitamin D helps your body absorb calcium and supports your immune system. It's especially important during pregnancy to ensure that your baby's bones develop properly. Aim for about 600 IU of vitamin D daily, which can be obtained from sunlight and fatty fish like salmon.

7. Fiber

Fiber is important for digestion, and many pregnant women experience constipation. Eating enough fiber can help prevent or ease this discomfort. High-fiber foods include whole grains, fruits, vegetables, and legumes.

How to Balance Calorie Intake with Nutrient Needs

With all of these nutrients to consider, it can feel overwhelming trying to figure out how to balance your calories. Here's how to approach it:

1. Eat a Variety of Nutrient-Dense Foods

Focus on whole foods that are rich in vitamins, minerals, and other essential nutrients. Include plenty of fruits, vegetables, lean proteins, whole grains, and healthy fats in your diet. Aim to eat a variety of colors on your plate to ensure you're getting a wide range of nutrients.

2. Choose Whole Grains Over Refined Carbs

While you'll need extra calories during pregnancy, the source of those calories matters. Choose whole grains like brown rice, oats, quinoa, and whole wheat bread over refined carbohydrates like white bread and pasta.

3. Snack Smartly

If you find yourself hungry between meals, choose healthy snacks that combine protein, fiber, and healthy fats. Examples include a handful of nuts and dried fruit, a slice of whole-grain toast with avocado, or a yogurt parfait with fresh fruit and granola. Avoid sugary snacks, as they can lead to unhealthy weight gain and blood sugar spikes.

4. Limit Empty-Calorie Foods

It can be tempting to indulge in high-calorie, low-nutrient foods during pregnancy (think cookies, chips, and sugary drinks), but it's important to limit these foods. While it's fine to have an occasional treat, try not to make them a regular part of your diet. These foods provide extra calories but little nutritional value, which could cause unhealthy weight gain or lead to nutrient deficiencies.

5. Hydration is Key

Drinking enough water is essential during pregnancy. Staying hydrated helps prevent dehydration and supports the increase in blood volume that occurs during pregnancy. Water also helps in digestion and can aid in preventing constipation. Try to drink at least 8-10 cups of water daily, more if you are active or the weather is hot.

Conclusion

Balancing nutrient intake with calorie needs is crucial during pregnancy. Focus on nutrient-dense foods, listen to your body's hunger cues, and avoid empty-calorie foods to support both your health and your baby's development. With mindful eating, you can ensure that you're nourishing yourself with the right balance of nutrients to help you feel your best throughout your pregnancy.

Strategic Suggestions

- **Eat small meals frequently** throughout the day to maintain your energy and prevent overeating at mealtimes.

- **Plan meals ahead** to ensure you're getting a balance of proteins, healthy fats, and fiber with every meal.

- **Incorporate a variety of fruits and vegetables** into your meals for essential vitamins, minerals, and fiber.

- **Limit processed snacks and sugary foods**, which provide empty calories without the nutrients your body needs.

- **Monitor your weight gain and adjust your food choices** as needed. Consult your healthcare provider to ensure your nutritional needs are being met.

Postpartum Weight Loss: Setting Realistic Goals

After giving birth, many new mothers are eager to return to their pre-pregnancy bodies. While it's understandable to want to regain your shape, it's essential to approach postpartum weight loss with patience, mindfulness, and realistic expectations. This is a time for nurturing both your physical and mental well-being, and losing weight should not be rushed. Let's break down a healthy approach to postpartum weight loss, keeping in mind that every woman's experience is unique.

Understanding Postpartum Weight Loss

Immediately after birth, your body naturally sheds a portion of the weight from pregnancy. You'll lose about 10 to 12 pounds right away, including the weight of the baby, placenta, and amniotic fluid. Over the next few weeks and months, your body will continue to adjust. However, it's important to keep in mind that it's not uncommon for weight loss to be slower than you might expect. Your body needs time to heal and regain strength, and it's not ideal to set too aggressive goals too early.

The timeline for postpartum weight loss can vary greatly, depending on factors such as genetics, the amount of weight you gained during pregnancy, your activity level, and if you are breastfeeding. On average, most women can expect to lose about 1 to 2 pounds per month over the first six months after giving birth. After that, the weight loss may slow down as your body adjusts. Focus on making steady, sustainable changes rather than aiming for rapid weight loss.

Factors That Affect Postpartum Weight Loss

Several factors can influence how quickly or slowly you lose weight after childbirth. Understanding these factors can help set realistic goals for yourself.

1. Breastfeeding

Breastfeeding can aid in postpartum weight loss. When you breastfeed, your body burns extra calories (about 300 to 500 calories per day) to produce milk. This can help you lose weight gradually over time. However, don't focus solely on breastfeeding as a quick fix for weight loss. It's essential to maintain a balanced diet while breastfeeding to ensure you're still meeting your nutritional needs and your baby's needs.

2. Sleep and Stress

Lack of sleep and high stress can hinder weight loss. New parents often experience sleep deprivation, which can lead to imbalances in hunger hormones, making it more difficult to control cravings. Chronic stress can also contribute to weight retention, particularly in the abdominal area. Try to manage stress, getting as much rest as possible, asking for help when needed, and practicing relaxation techniques like deep breathing or meditation.

3. Physical Activity

Engaging in regular physical activity is one of the best ways to boost postpartum weight loss. However, it's essential to ease back into exercise after childbirth, especially if you had a cesarean section or any complications. Start with gentle exercises like walking or postpartum yoga, and gradually increase the intensity as your body heals. Consult your healthcare provider before starting any exercise regimen, particularly if you have any concerns about your recovery.

4. Diet and Nutrition

While breastfeeding and exercise contribute to weight loss, your diet plays a significant role. Aim for a nutrient-dense, balanced diet that includes plenty of whole grains, lean proteins, healthy fats, and vegetables. It's important to avoid overly restrictive diets, as they can affect your energy levels, milk supply, and overall health. Instead, focus on portion control and making healthier food choices.

Setting Realistic Goals for Postpartum Weight Loss

Setting realistic and achievable goals for postpartum weight loss is important for your physical and emotional health. Here's how to set yourself up for success:

1. Start Slow and Be Patient

It's easy to feel frustrated if you don't see immediate results, but slow and steady weight loss is more sustainable. Give yourself at least 6 weeks to recover before starting a weight loss plan, and even then, aim for losing no more than 1-2 pounds per week. This gives your body time to heal and adjust, and it also ensures that the weight you lose is primarily fat rather than muscle or water.

2. Focus on Overall Health, Not Just Weight

Rather than obsessing over a specific number on the scale, shift your focus to how you feel and how your body is functioning. Celebrate non-scale victories like improved energy levels, better sleep, or fitting into clothes more comfortably. These signs are just as important as weight loss and reflect your overall well-being.

3. Track Your Progress

Keeping track of your progress can help you stay motivated, but avoid fixating solely on the scale. Consider tracking other measurements such as your body measurements, how your clothes fit, and how much physical activity you're getting each week. Write down how you feel—emotionally and physically—as this can help you focus on the holistic nature of your health and not just the number on the scale.

4. Set SMART Goals

Setting SMART (Specific, Measurable, Achievable, Relevant, and Time-bound) goals can help you create clear, actionable steps toward postpartum weight loss. For example, rather than setting a vague goal of "lose weight," a SMART goal might be "Walk for 30 minutes every day for the next two weeks" or "Eat three balanced meals and two snacks each day for the next month." This gives you clear objectives to work toward and helps you stay motivated along the way.

5. Celebrate Small Wins

The postpartum period can feel overwhelming, and weight loss can sometimes take longer than anticipated. It's important to acknowledge and celebrate small wins along the way, such as completing a workout, making healthier food choices, or simply getting more sleep. These small steps build up over time and contribute to a healthier lifestyle.

6. Seek Support and Guidance

Having a support system during the postpartum period is crucial. This can be in the form of family, friends, or a professional, like a dietitian or personal trainer. If you're struggling with body image issues or feeling overwhelmed with weight loss pressure, speaking with a healthcare provider can provide reassurance and helpful advice.

Conclusion

Postpartum weight loss is not a race. It's a process that should be approached with patience and realistic goals. Prioritize overall health, focus on sustainable habits, and give yourself the grace to recover from childbirth at your own pace. Set small, achievable goals and be kind to yourself to navigate this phase with confidence and well-being.

Strategic Suggestions

- **Take it slow and focus on gradual changes** to avoid overwhelming yourself.
- **Incorporate exercise slowly**, and be sure to consult your healthcare provider before resuming physical activity.
- **Prioritize balanced meals** to fuel your body and support breastfeeding.

- **Avoid restrictive diets** that could harm your milk supply or energy levels.

- **Focus on mental health** to manage stress and getting enough sleep are essential components of weight loss.

- **Track progress beyond the scale** to celebrate improvements in overall health and energy.

Chapter 9: Supporting Mental and Emotional Well-Being Through Diet

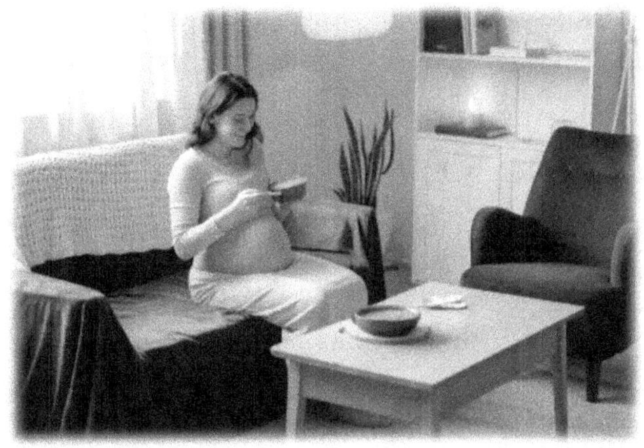

Supporting mental and emotional well-being during pregnancy is crucial for both your health and your baby's development. A balanced diet rich in specific nutrients can help stabilize mood, reduce stress, and improve emotional resilience. Proper nutrition plays an essential role in fostering a positive pregnancy experience.

The Connection Between Food and Mood

During pregnancy, it's common to experience shifts in mood, ranging from joy to anxiety, excitement to irritability. But did you know that what you eat can influence how you feel emotionally? The connection between food and mood is not just a passing idea—it's rooted in science. Many pregnant women find that their emotions are closely tied to the nutrients they consume, the changes in their body, and the hormonal fluctuations that come with pregnancy. As a result, understanding how food impacts your mood can help you maintain emotional stability and improve your overall well-being.

A balanced diet during pregnancy is essential not only for physical health but also for emotional health. It is well-known that food affects brain chemistry, and certain nutrients are directly linked to the production of mood-regulating neurotransmitters such as serotonin and dopamine. These neurotransmitters help regulate feelings of happiness, calmness, and overall emotional well-being. A diet rich in vitamins, minerals, and healthy fats can enhance brain function and help maintain mood balance throughout pregnancy.

The Science Behind Food and Mood

Your brain relies on specific nutrients to function properly. For example, Omega-3 fatty acids, found in fish like salmon and in flaxseeds, are essential for brain health and have been linked to improved mood and mental clarity. Studies suggest that pregnant women who are deficient in Omega-3 fatty acids may experience higher levels of anxiety and depression. Adding these healthy fats to your diet can have a positive impact on your mood.

Another key nutrient is folic acid, which is vital during pregnancy, especially in the early stages. Folic acid plays a crucial role in the production of serotonin, the "feel-good" neurotransmitter. Serotonin is important for regulating mood, sleep, and appetite. A deficiency in folic acid during pregnancy has been associated with an increased risk of mood disorders, such as depression and anxiety. Incorporating folic acid-rich foods, like leafy greens, beans, and fortified cereals, into your diet can support your mental health.

Protein is another nutrient that plays a significant role in mood regulation. Amino acids, the building blocks of protein, are essential for the production of neurotransmitters. A steady intake of protein throughout the day helps maintain stable blood sugar levels, preventing the irritability and fatigue that often accompany mood swings.

The Role of Gut Health in Emotional Balance

The gut is sometimes referred to as the "second brain" because of its role in producing neurotransmitters. In fact, about 95% of serotonin is produced in the gut. This means that the health of your digestive system plays a big role in how you feel emotionally. A healthy gut microbiome—comprised of billions of bacteria—supports the production of serotonin and other brain chemicals that influence mood.

Eating a diet rich in fiber, probiotics, and prebiotics can promote a healthy gut microbiome. Fiber-rich foods, like whole grains, fruits, and vegetables, help feed the beneficial bacteria in your gut. Probiotics, found in fermented foods such as yogurt, kefir, and kimchi, support gut health, as they introduce beneficial bacteria. Prebiotics, found in foods like garlic, onions, and bananas, nourish these bacteria and help them thrive.

Blood Sugar Balance and Mood Swings

One of the most common emotional challenges during pregnancy is mood swings, which are often triggered by fluctuations in blood sugar levels. When your blood sugar drops too low, you may feel irritable, anxious, or fatigued. Conversely, when blood sugar spikes, you might feel jittery or overly energetic. Maintaining stable blood sugar levels throughout the day can help prevent these mood swings and keep your energy levels consistent.

To maintain balanced blood sugar, try eating smaller, more frequent meals that combine protein, healthy fats, and fiber. For example, a snack of apple slices with almond butter provides fiber, healthy fats, and protein—all of which help stabilize blood sugar. Avoid sugary snacks and refined carbohydrates, which can cause blood sugar spikes, then crashes, leading to mood fluctuations.

Hydration and Emotional Well-being

Staying hydrated is just as important for your mood as eating the right foods. Dehydration can contribute to feelings of irritability, fatigue, and even anxiety. During pregnancy, your body's fluid needs increase, so it's essential to drink plenty of water throughout the day. Aim for at least 8–10 cups of water daily, and consider adding electrolyte-rich drinks like coconut water to replenish lost minerals.

Practical Tips for Improving Mood Through Diet

- **Include Omega-3s**

Add fatty fish like salmon or chia seeds to your meals to support brain health and mood regulation.

- **Focus on Protein**

Incorporate lean proteins such as chicken, eggs, or legumes in your meals to stabilize blood sugar and support neurotransmitter production.

- **Consume Folate-Rich Foods**

Incorporating leafy greens, beans, and fortified cereals into your diet is a powerful way to support serotonin production and maintain emotional balance. Serotonin is a neurotransmitter often referred to as the "feel-good" chemical because it helps regulate mood, appetite, and sleep.

- **Stay Hydrated**

Drink enough water and consume electrolyte-rich drinks to avoid dehydration, which can affect mood.

- **Support Gut Health**

Eat fiber-rich foods, and consider adding fermented foods like yogurt or kefir to your diet to enhance gut health and serotonin production.

Strategic Suggestions

To maintain a balanced mood throughout pregnancy, focus on eating whole, nutrient-dense foods, staying hydrated, and managing blood sugar levels. Incorporate foods that support brain health and gut health, and aim to eat balanced meals throughout the day. If mood swings or anxiety become overwhelming, talk to your healthcare provider about nutritional supplements or other interventions that might help.

Eating to Combat Pregnancy-Related Anxiety and Stress

Pregnancy is a time of profound change, both physically and emotionally. As you navigate these changes, it's common to experience feelings of anxiety and stress. Hormonal fluctuations, changes in your body, and the anticipation of becoming a parent can all contribute to emotional tension. While stress and anxiety are natural parts of pregnancy, the good news is that your diet can play a significant role in helping you manage these emotions. Make intentional food choices to help soothe your mind, support your emotional health, and reduce stress levels during this transformative time.

The Link Between Diet and Anxiety

Many foods have the potential to impact the way your body responds to stress. When you're anxious or stressed, your body produces higher levels of stress hormones like cortisol. Over time, high cortisol levels can affect your mood, energy, and even your immune system. On the other hand, certain foods can help reduce stress hormones and promote the production of neurotransmitters like serotonin and dopamine, which improve mood and relaxation.

The key to managing stress through diet lies in consuming nutrient-dense foods that support your body's ability to respond to and manage stress. Nutrients like magnesium, vitamin B6, Omega-3 fatty acids, and antioxidants all play a role in balancing your stress response and keeping your nervous system calm. Let's take a closer look at how specific foods and nutrients can help.

1. Magnesium for Stress Relief

Magnesium is often referred to as the "anti-stress mineral" because it plays a vital role in regulating your body's stress response. It helps relax muscles, calm the nervous system, and regulate cortisol levels. During pregnancy, magnesium also supports the development of your baby's bones and organs. A magnesium deficiency can contribute to symptoms of anxiety and irritability, which can make stress feel even more overwhelming.

Good sources of magnesium include leafy green vegetables like spinach and kale, nuts and seeds (especially almonds, sunflower seeds, and pumpkin seeds), whole grains like quinoa and brown rice, and legumes like beans and lentils. Aim to include magnesium-rich foods in your meals to help manage your anxiety levels and support your overall well-being.

2. Omega-3 Fatty Acids: Brain Health and Mood Regulation

Omega-3 fatty acids are essential fats that have been shown to have a positive impact on mental health. Research suggests that Omega-3s, found in fatty fish like salmon, sardines, and mackerel, as well as plant-based sources like flaxseeds, chia seeds, and walnuts, can help reduce symptoms of depression and anxiety.

Omega-3 fatty acids are important for brain function and the production of neurotransmitters that regulate mood. They help reduce inflammation in the brain and body, which can be particularly beneficial during pregnancy, as hormonal changes can sometimes lead to increased stress and anxiety. Incorporate more Omega-3-rich foods into your diet to support both your mental and physical health during this time.

3. Vitamin B6: Supporting Your Nervous System

Vitamin B6, or pyridoxine, plays a crucial role in the production of serotonin, the "feel-good" neurotransmitter that helps regulate mood and reduce feelings of anxiety. During pregnancy, your body's need for vitamin B6 increases, as it supports the development of your baby's nervous system and promotes healthy brain function. Low levels of B6 have been linked to increased anxiety and depression, making it particularly important to ensure you are getting enough during this time.

Vitamin B6 can be found in a variety of foods, including bananas, chickpeas, potatoes, poultry, and fortified cereals. If you're struggling with stress or anxiety, try to incorporate more of these foods into your diet to help balance your mood and promote a sense of calm.

4. Complex Carbohydrates for Stable Blood Sugar

Blood sugar imbalances can contribute to feelings of irritability and anxiety. Consuming too many refined carbohydrates or sugary foods can cause rapid spikes in blood sugar and crashes that leave you feeling jittery and on edge. On the other hand, complex carbohydrates, like those found in whole grains, fruits, and vegetables, release sugar slowly into your bloodstream, helping to maintain stable energy levels and prevent mood swings.

To keep your blood sugar stable and reduce anxiety, opt for whole grains like oats, quinoa, and brown rice, as well as fruits and vegetables that are high in fiber, such as berries, apples, and leafy greens. Pairing complex carbs with protein and healthy fats—such as a handful of nuts or avocado—can further help balance blood sugar levels and keep you feeling calm and energized throughout the day.

Hydration and Stress Management

Dehydration is often overlooked, but it can have a significant impact on your mood. When you're dehydrated, your body is more likely to respond to stress with higher levels of anxiety and irritability. During pregnancy, your hydration needs increase, and not drinking enough water can leave you feeling exhausted and overwhelmed. Aim to drink at least 8-10 cups of water a day, and consider adding hydrating foods like cucumbers, watermelon, and oranges to your meals and snacks.

Practical Tips for Eating to Manage Anxiety

- **Incorporate Magnesium-Rich Foods**

Incorporating leafy greens, nuts, seeds, and whole grains into your diet can be an excellent way to help relax your nervous system and promote emotional balance.

- **Add Omega-3 Fatty Acids**

Include fatty fish like salmon, chia seeds, and flaxseeds to support brain health and reduce anxiety.

- **Boost Your Vitamin B6 Intake**

Eat bananas, chickpeas, and poultry to help regulate serotonin levels and improve mood.

- **Opt for Complex Carbs**

Choose whole grains, fruits, and vegetables to maintain stable blood sugar levels and prevent mood swings.

- **Stay Hydrated**

Drink plenty of water and eat water-rich foods like fruits and vegetables to avoid dehydration, which can exacerbate anxiety.

Strategic Suggestions

To manage pregnancy-related anxiety and stress, focus on a balanced diet that includes magnesium-rich foods, Omega-3s, vitamin B6, and complex carbohydrates. Aim to stay hydrated and include foods that support your nervous system and overall well-being. If you're struggling with anxiety, consult with your healthcare provider about further strategies, such as relaxation techniques or therapy, that can help support your emotional health during pregnancy.

Comfort Foods That Support Mental Health

Pregnancy is a time of great emotional and physical change, and it's only natural to crave comfort foods during this period. Comfort foods are often associated with feelings of warmth, security, and relaxation, which can be especially helpful when you're navigating the emotional ups and downs that come with pregnancy. However, the challenge lies in choosing comfort foods that not only satisfy cravings but also provide nourishment and support your mental health. Thankfully, many comfort foods can be both delicious and beneficial for your emotional well-being, helping you manage stress, anxiety, and other mood-related challenges.

Why Comfort Foods Matter During Pregnancy

The connection between food and mood is not just anecdotal. Certain foods can actually impact the chemicals in your brain that regulate mood and emotion. When you're pregnant, you're already dealing with a lot of physical and emotional stress due to fluctuating hormones and the anticipation of parenthood. Comfort foods can help reduce stress and improve mood when chosen wisely, providing the brain with nutrients it needs to maintain balance and calm.

Comfort foods can also provide a sense of familiarity and nostalgia, which can be soothing during times of uncertainty or stress. This emotional connection can help reduce anxiety and create a feeling of stability. However, it's essential to choose comfort foods that nourish both your body and mind.

Nutrient-Dense Comfort Foods for Mental Health

1. Oats and Whole Grains

Oats, quinoa, and other whole grains are excellent choices when you're craving a hearty, comforting meal. These foods are rich in complex carbohydrates, which are key for maintaining stable blood sugar levels. Stable blood sugar levels are crucial for emotional balance, as fluctuations in blood sugar can lead to irritability, fatigue, and mood swings. Whole grains also contain B vitamins, which are essential for nervous system health and help regulate mood. Oats, in particular, contain tryptophan, an amino acid that the body uses to produce serotonin—the neurotransmitter that promotes feelings of happiness and well-being.

Try incorporating oatmeal into your breakfast routine, adding toppings like berries, nuts, and seeds for extra fiber, protein, and healthy fats. You can also experiment with whole-grain muffins, pancakes, or quinoa salads for lunch or dinner.

2. Avocado: The Creamy, Comforting Superfood

Avocados are another comfort food that can support both your emotional and physical health. Rich in healthy monounsaturated fats, avocados help regulate your brain's neurotransmitters, supporting a calm, stable mood. They also contain folate, which is important for both your mental health and your baby's development. Folate has been shown to reduce the risk of depression and anxiety during pregnancy, and avocados are one of the best natural sources of this vital nutrient.

You can enjoy avocado as a topping for toast, in a creamy guacamole, or even blended into a smoothie. The creamy texture can be especially comforting, and the nutrients will help nourish your body and mind.

3. Dark Chocolate: A Sweet Mood Booster

Craving something sweet? Dark chocolate, particularly varieties with at least 70% cocoa, can be a beneficial comfort food during pregnancy. Dark chocolate contains magnesium, which helps relax your muscles and calm your nervous system. It also boosts serotonin levels, which can help elevate mood and reduce stress. Furthermore, dark chocolate is rich in antioxidants, which can help combat inflammation and support overall health.

You don't have to indulge in large quantities to reap the benefits. A small piece of dark chocolate, perhaps with a handful of almonds, can be a satisfying and mood-boosting treat. Pairing it with other brain-boosting foods, such as walnuts, can amplify the positive effects on your mood.

4. Berries and Fresh Fruit

When you're craving something refreshing, fresh fruit—especially berries—can be a great option. Berries like strawberries, blueberries, and raspberries are packed with antioxidants, which can help reduce stress and combat the effects of oxidative stress in the body. They are also high in vitamin C, which supports the immune system and has been linked to reduced levels of anxiety and stress.

You can enjoy berries on their own, add them to yogurt or oatmeal, or even blend them into smoothies. For a comforting dessert, try a berry compote with a drizzle of honey or a few pieces of dark chocolate.

5. Nuts and Seeds

Nuts and seeds, such as almonds, walnuts, chia seeds, and flaxseeds, are small yet powerful comfort foods for mental health. These foods are high in Omega-3 fatty acids, which help reduce inflammation in the brain and improve mood. Walnuts, in particular, are rich in tryptophan, which helps produce serotonin, the "feel-good" neurotransmitter. Nuts and seeds also contain magnesium, which helps alleviate feelings of anxiety and stress.

Snacking on a handful of mixed nuts or adding them to your oatmeal or salads can provide sustained energy and keep your mood stable. They also make great additions to baked goods like muffins or granola bars.

6. Soup and Stews: Warmth and Comfort

A warm bowl of soup or stew can be incredibly comforting, especially during cooler months. Bone broth-based soups are packed with nutrients like collagen, which supports your skin and joints during pregnancy, and amino acids like glycine, which promote relaxation and better sleep. Vegetables like carrots, sweet potatoes, and leafy greens in soups provide vital nutrients like vitamin A, potassium, and magnesium, all of which support your mental and emotional well-being.

Homemade soups can be a wonderful way to load up on nourishing vegetables and feel comforted at the same time. You can make large batches and store them in the fridge or freezer for quick, easy access during busy days.

Making Comfort Foods Part of a Balanced Diet

While comfort foods are a great way to manage stress and promote mental health during pregnancy, it's important to keep them balanced with a variety of other nutrient-dense foods. These comfort foods should be part of a well-rounded diet that includes plenty of vegetables, lean proteins, whole grains, and healthy fats. Also, remember that comfort foods should be enjoyed in moderation, especially when they contain higher amounts of sugar or salt.

Strategic Suggestions

To use comfort foods effectively for mental well-being during pregnancy, focus on foods that nourish the body and mind, such as whole grains, avocados, dark chocolate, fresh fruits, and nuts. Aim to balance your cravings with healthy options that support mood stability and emotional health. Always listen to your body and make adjustments as needed to maintain both your physical and mental well-being.

Chapter 10: Meal Planning and Recipes for Pregnant Mothers

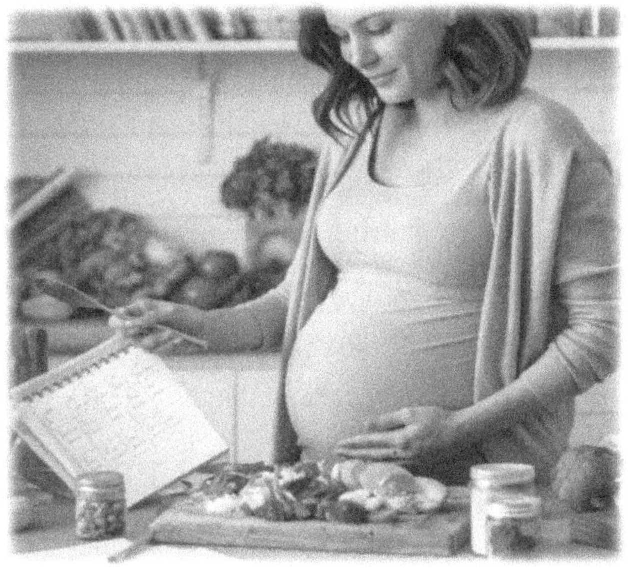

Meal planning during pregnancy is essential for ensuring both you and your baby receive optimal nutrition. Creating balanced, nutrient-dense meals helps manage hunger, supports your baby's development, and maintains your energy levels throughout the day. Planning ahead can simplify mealtime while meeting your nutritional needs.

Building a Weekly Meal Plan for Pregnancy

Pregnancy is an exciting time, but it can also be overwhelming, especially when it comes to meal planning. Eating a well-balanced diet is essential to support both your health and your baby's development. A weekly meal plan can help reduce stress around meal times and ensure you're getting all the nutrients you need. Carefully organize your meals to avoid unhealthy choices, save time, and maintain a consistent, nutrient-packed diet.

The Importance of Meal Planning During Pregnancy

When you're pregnant, your body has higher nutritional demands. You're not just eating for yourself, but for your growing baby. A carefully crafted meal plan ensures that you're getting the right balance of proteins, vitamins, minerals, healthy fats, and carbohydrates to support pregnancy. The right foods can help with energy levels, mood stability, and fetal development.

Additionally, meal planning allows you to make informed decisions about your food choices. It can help you meet your daily requirements for critical nutrients like folate, iron, calcium, and omega-3 fatty acids. Consistently eating healthy meals will also help you avoid the temptation to grab convenience foods, which may not always provide the essential nutrients you need.

Steps to Build a Weekly Meal Plan for Pregnancy

1. Assess Your Nutritional Needs

Before starting your meal plan, it's important to understand the nutrients you need during pregnancy. Some of the most important nutrients include:

- **Folate (Vitamin B9):** Crucial for preventing neural tube defects and supporting cell division.

- **Iron:** Important for increasing blood volume and preventing anemia.
- **Calcium:** Helps build your baby's bones and teeth.
- **Protein:** Essential for tissue growth and fetal development.
- **Healthy fats:** Important for brain development and hormonal regulation.

Ensure that your weekly plan includes a variety of foods rich in these nutrients, such as leafy greens, fortified cereals, dairy products, lean meats, eggs, beans, nuts, and seeds.

2. Plan Balanced Meals

Each meal should include a balance of protein, healthy fats, and complex carbohydrates to keep you feeling satisfied and energized. For instance, a well-balanced lunch might consist of:

- **Protein:** Grilled chicken or tofu
- **Healthy Fats:** A side of avocado or olive oil-based dressing

- **Carbohydrates:** Brown rice or sweet potatoes

- **Veggies:** A colorful salad or steamed broccoli This combination helps ensure you're not only full but also nourishing your body with the right macronutrients.

3. Incorporate Pregnancy Superfoods

There are certain foods that are especially beneficial during pregnancy, often referred to as "superfoods." These include:

- **Leafy greens:** High in folate, iron, and calcium.

- **Fatty fish:** Rich in omega-3 fatty acids for brain development.

- **Eggs:** A great source of protein, choline, and other vital vitamins.

- **Berries:** Packed with antioxidants and vitamin C for immune support.

- **Nuts and seeds:** Good sources of healthy fats and protein.

Make sure to include these superfoods in your meal plan at least a few times a week to maximize the health benefits for both you and your baby.

Create a Grocery List

Once you've mapped out your meals for the week, create a shopping list based on your plan. This helps you avoid impulse buys and ensures you only purchase the ingredients you need. Consider shopping in bulk for pantry staples like oats, quinoa, beans, and lentils, which can be used in multiple meals. Fresh produce and protein sources should be bought weekly to ensure they're fresh.

Prep Meals in Advance

Meal prep can be a lifesaver during pregnancy, especially when you're feeling tired or nauseous. Preparing meals in advance or even just chopping vegetables and marinating proteins ahead of time can save you hours during the week. You can batch-cook soups, casseroles, or grains, so all you have to do is reheat them when you're hungry. Consider investing in good-quality containers to store prepped meals in the fridge or freezer.

Include Healthy Snacks

Pregnancy often comes with increased hunger or cravings, so it's helpful to plan for snacks that are both nutritious and satisfying. Stock your kitchen with:

- Greek yogurt with nuts or berries
- Sliced veggies with hummus
- Whole-grain crackers with cheese
- A small handful of mixed nuts

Fresh fruit or a smoothie with spinach, banana, and almond milk These snacks can help keep your energy up and prevent unhealthy snacking.

Adjust for Dietary Restrictions or Preferences

If you have any dietary restrictions, such as being vegetarian or gluten-free, adjust your meal plan accordingly. For instance, if you're vegetarian, include plant-based proteins like lentils, chickpeas, tofu, and quinoa. If you need to avoid dairy, try plant-based milk and calcium-rich non-dairy options like fortified almond milk or leafy greens. The key is to focus on nutrient-dense foods, regardless of dietary preferences.

Strategic Suggestions

- **Prep Ingredients, Not Just Meals:** If cooking full meals in advance feels overwhelming, try prepping individual ingredients (e.g., chopping vegetables or cooking grains) and assembling meals as needed.

- **Stay Flexible:** Life during pregnancy can be unpredictable, so build flexibility into your meal plan. Keep easy-to-make meals on hand for busy days.

- **Use a Meal Planning App:** If you're tech-savvy, try using an app or online meal planner to organize your meals, create shopping lists, and find new recipe ideas.

Follow these steps and strategies to create a meal plan that will nourish you and your baby while taking some of the stress out of pregnancy.

Quick and Easy Recipes for Busy Moms-to-Be

Pregnancy is a time when your body's nutritional needs are at an all-time high. But with all the changes, fatigue, and busy schedules, it's not always easy to prioritize healthy eating. The good news is that there are plenty of quick and easy recipes that will nourish both you and your baby while fitting into a busy lifestyle. If you're dealing with pregnancy-related fatigue, nausea, or simply don't have the energy to spend hours in the kitchen, these recipes can help you get the nutrients you need in a fraction of the time.

Why Quick and Easy Meals Matter During Pregnancy

In pregnancy, your body requires more energy and nutrients to support both your health and your baby's development. However, the increased fatigue and time constraints can make meal planning seem daunting. Quick, easy recipes are essential because they allow you to stay on top of your nutritional needs without feeling overwhelmed.

These meals can help manage common pregnancy symptoms like nausea or cravings and can support your immune system, energy levels, and overall well-being. Plus, they can ensure you're consistently consuming a variety of vitamins, minerals, and macronutrients—critical for your baby's growth and development.

Quick and Easy Recipes for Busy Moms-to-Be

1. One-Pan Veggie and Chicken Stir-Fry

This simple and versatile recipe can be adapted to suit your tastes. It's loaded with protein, fiber, and healthy fats to fuel you throughout the day.

Ingredients:

- 1 lb chicken breast or thighs, sliced into strips

- 2 cups mixed vegetables (broccoli, bell peppers, carrots)
- 1 tablespoon olive oil
- 2 tablespoons soy sauce (or tamari for gluten-free)
- 1 teaspoon ginger (optional)
- 1 tablespoon garlic, minced
- Cooked brown rice (optional)

Instructions:

- Heat olive oil in a large pan over medium heat. Add the chicken and cook until browned, about 5-7 minutes.
- Add the garlic, ginger, and mixed vegetables to the pan, stirring occasionally.
- Once the vegetables are tender, pour in the soy sauce and stir until everything is well-coated.
- Serve with brown rice for a complete meal.

This recipe is quick, provides lean protein, and offers a healthy balance of vegetables and whole grains. If you prefer a vegetarian version, swap the chicken for tofu or chickpeas.

2. Quick Breakfast Smoothie

Smoothies are one of the easiest ways to pack a lot of nutrients into one meal. They're great for mornings when you're rushed or when you have trouble eating solid food due to nausea or other pregnancy symptoms.

Ingredients:

- 1 banana
- 1 cup spinach (fresh or frozen)
- 1 tablespoon peanut butter or almond butter
- 1/2 cup plain Greek yogurt
- 1/2 cup almond milk (or any milk of choice)
- 1 tablespoon chia seeds or flaxseeds

Instructions:

- Add all ingredients to a blender and blend until smooth.
- Adjust the consistency with more milk if needed.

This smoothie is packed with folate from the spinach, healthy fats from the peanut butter and seeds, and protein from Greek yogurt. It's a great way to get a nutritious start to your day, especially if you're struggling with morning sickness or fatigue.

3. Simple Avocado Toast with Eggs

Avocado toast is not only trendy but also packed with nutrients for pregnancy. The healthy fats from the avocado and the protein from the eggs make this meal both satisfying and filling.

Ingredients:

- 1 ripe avocado
- 2 slices of whole-grain or gluten-free bread
- 2 eggs (scrambled or fried)

- Salt and pepper, to taste
- Chili flakes (optional)

Instructions:

- Toast the bread to your liking.
- While the bread is toasting, mash the avocado with a fork, adding salt, pepper, and chili flakes for extra flavor.
- Cook the eggs to your preference.
- Spread the mashed avocado onto the toast and top with the eggs.

This meal is high in fiber, healthy fats, and protein, making it an excellent option for a quick breakfast or light lunch.

3. Vegetable and Bean Chili

A hearty vegetable chili is a nutrient-dense option that can be prepared in under 30 minutes. Beans provide plant-based protein and fiber, while the tomatoes, peppers, and onions provide essential vitamins and minerals.

Ingredients:

- 1 can kidney beans, drained and rinsed
- 1 can black beans, drained and rinsed
- 1 can diced tomatoes
- 1 bell pepper, chopped
- 1 onion, chopped
- 1 tablespoon olive oil
- 2 teaspoons chili powder
- 1/2 teaspoon cumin
- Salt and pepper to taste

Instructions:

- Heat the olive oil in a large pot over medium heat. Add the onion and bell pepper and sauté until soft, about 5 minutes.
- Add the chili powder, cumin, beans, and tomatoes. Stir well and bring to a simmer.
- Let it cook for 20-30 minutes, stirring occasionally. Add salt and pepper to taste.

This recipe can be made in one pot and is an excellent source of protein and fiber. You can add some shredded cheese or a dollop of sour cream for extra flavor.

4. Stuffed Sweet Potatoes

Sweet potatoes are a nutrient powerhouse, packed with beta-carotene and fiber. This easy meal can be topped with various toppings to suit your cravings.

Ingredients:

- 2 sweet potatoes
- 1/2 cup black beans, rinsed
- 1/4 cup Greek yogurt
- 1/4 cup shredded cheese (optional)
- Fresh cilantro, chopped

Instructions:

- Preheat your oven to 400°F (200°C). Pierce the sweet potatoes with a fork and bake them for 30-40 minutes, until tender.

- While they bake, heat the black beans on the stove or in the microwave.
- Once the sweet potatoes are done, slice them open and fluff the insides with a fork.
- Top with black beans, Greek yogurt, cheese, and cilantro.

These stuffed sweet potatoes are a delicious, quick way to enjoy a balanced meal that's rich in fiber and protein.

Strategic Suggestions

- **Batch Cook and Freeze:** Whenever you have time, make larger batches of your favorite recipes and freeze them. This will give you quick, ready-made meals when you're too tired to cook.
- **Keep Healthy Ingredients on Hand:** Stock up on easy-to-use ingredients like canned beans, frozen vegetables, whole grains, and pre-

cooked chicken. These staples make it easy to throw together a nutritious meal in minutes.

- **Mix Up Simple Recipes:** Even simple meals can feel new if you change up the spices, add different toppings, or swap out a vegetable or protein.

With these quick and easy recipes, you can nourish your body during pregnancy without spending hours in the kitchen. Keep your meals balanced, nutritious, and enjoyable, and you'll be well on your way to supporting both your and your baby's health.

Snacks and Smoothies Packed with Nutrients

During pregnancy, it's essential to nourish your body with nutrient-dense foods throughout the day. While meals provide the bulk of your daily nutrition, snacks and smoothies are an excellent way to fill in the gaps, keep your energy levels up, and ensure you're getting the vitamins and minerals both you and your baby need. These snacks and smoothies are easy to make, portable, and offer a great variety of nutrients, making them ideal for busy moms-to-be.

The Importance of Snacks and Smoothies During Pregnancy

Pregnancy can cause increased hunger, and many women experience fluctuations in their energy levels, especially in the first and third trimesters. Snacking on healthy foods can help you manage your appetite, stabilize blood sugar levels, and keep your energy steady throughout the day. Healthy snacks and smoothies are also a great way to make sure you're meeting your increased nutrient requirements, especially for essential vitamins and minerals like folate, iron, calcium, and protein.

When choosing snacks and smoothies during pregnancy, focus on options that are rich in nutrients rather than empty calories. Choose foods that will provide lasting energy, help your body heal, and support your growing baby's development. Snacks and smoothies that combine protein, healthy fats, and complex carbohydrates will leave you feeling satisfied and less likely to overeat later.

Nutrient-Rich Snack Ideas for Pregnant Women

1. Greek Yogurt Parfait with Berries and Nuts

Greek yogurt is a fantastic source of calcium and protein, both of which are vital during pregnancy. Paired with fiber-rich berries and heart-healthy nuts, this snack provides a powerful nutritional punch.

Ingredients:

- 1 cup plain Greek yogurt
- 1/4 cup mixed berries (blueberries, strawberries, raspberries)
- 1 tablespoon chopped almonds or walnuts
- 1 teaspoon honey (optional)

Instructions:

- Layer the Greek yogurt and berries in a bowl or jar.
- Top with chopped nuts and drizzle with honey for extra sweetness.
- Enjoy as a quick and nutritious snack.

This parfait is an excellent source of calcium, protein, and antioxidants. You can vary the fruit depending on the season.

2. Hummus with Veggies or Whole Grain Crackers

Hummus is a protein-packed snack made from chickpeas, and it's perfect for pairing with crunchy veggies like carrots, cucumber, or bell peppers. If you're craving something heartier, whole grain crackers can also make a great accompaniment.

Ingredients:

- 1/4 cup hummus
- 1/2 cup baby carrots, cucumber slices, or bell pepper strips
- 5-6 whole grain crackers

Instructions:

- Dip your vegetables or crackers into the hummus.
- Enjoy as a satisfying snack rich in fiber, healthy fats, and protein.

This snack is an excellent choice if you want something that will keep you full, as it combines protein, fiber, and healthy fats. The fiber in the veggies and the healthy fats in the hummus help maintain blood sugar levels and provide lasting energy.

3. Hard-Boiled Eggs with Avocado

Eggs are packed with protein, vitamin D, and healthy fats—key nutrients during pregnancy. Paired with avocado, which is rich in folate, fiber, and healthy fats, this snack is both filling and nutritious.

Ingredients:

- 1-2 hard-boiled eggs
- 1/2 avocado, sliced
- A pinch of salt and pepper

Instructions:

- Peel the hard-boiled eggs and slice them.
- Mash or slice the avocado and spread it over the eggs.
- Season with salt and pepper, and enjoy.

This simple snack provides a great balance of protein, healthy fats, and fiber. It's especially helpful if you're craving something savory or need a protein boost in between meals.

4. Cottage Cheese with Pineapple and Chia Seeds

Cottage cheese is rich in protein and calcium, making it an excellent choice for pregnant women. Pairing it with pineapple, which is high in vitamin C, and chia seeds, which provide fiber and omega-3 fatty acids, creates a well-rounded and refreshing snack.

Ingredients:

- 1/2 cup cottage cheese
- 1/2 cup pineapple chunks
- 1 tablespoon chia seeds

Instructions:

- Combine the cottage cheese and pineapple in a bowl.
- Sprinkle the chia seeds on top and enjoy.

This snack is great for supporting your immune system, digestive health, and skin elasticity during pregnancy. The combination of protein, healthy fats, and fiber makes it both satisfying and nutrient-packed.

5. Apple Slices with Peanut Butter

Apples are high in fiber and vitamin C, while peanut butter adds protein and healthy fats. This snack is quick, satisfying, and perfect for a midday energy boost.

Ingredients:

- 1 apple, sliced
- 2 tablespoons natural peanut butter (or almond butter)

Instructions:

- Slice the apple and dip it into the peanut butter.
- Enjoy as a simple and filling snack.

The fiber from the apple helps with digestion, while the healthy fats and protein from the peanut butter keep you full longer. Make sure to choose a peanut butter without added sugar or unhealthy fats.

Nutrient-Dense Smoothies for Pregnancy

Smoothies are one of the best ways to pack in a lot of nutrients quickly, especially if you're struggling with nausea or fatigue. They're easily customizable and can include everything from fruits and vegetables to protein sources.

1. Green Pregnancy Smoothie

Packed with iron, folate, and vitamins, this smoothie is perfect for supporting your body's increasing nutritional needs.

Ingredients:

- 1 cup spinach or kale
- 1/2 banana
- 1/2 cup frozen mango or pineapple
- 1/2 cup Greek yogurt
- 1/2 cup unsweetened almond milk

Instructions:

- Blend all ingredients until smooth.
- Drink as a nutrient-rich snack.

This smoothie is rich in folate, iron, and calcium, essential for both you and your baby's development. The spinach or kale provides a serving of greens, while the yogurt adds a boost of protein and probiotics.

2. Berry Protein Smoothie

A great source of antioxidants, fiber, and protein, this smoothie helps to keep you full and energized.

Ingredients:

- 1 cup mixed berries (strawberries, blueberries, raspberries)
- 1/2 cup Greek yogurt
- 1 tablespoon chia seeds or flaxseeds
- 1/2 cup almond milk or any milk of your choice

Instructions:

- Blend all ingredients together until smooth.
- Pour into a glass and enjoy.

This smoothie is high in vitamin C, antioxidants, and protein, making it great for your immune system and overall health.

Strategic Suggestions

- **Plan Ahead:** Prepare snack portions in advance and store them in containers. Pre-chop fruits, veggies, or make smoothie packs so you can easily grab them when you're in a rush.

- **Combine Protein and Fiber:** Focus on snacks that contain a combination of protein and fiber. This combination helps you feel fuller for longer and stabilizes blood sugar levels.

- **Stay Hydrated:** Don't forget to drink plenty of water throughout the day. Staying hydrated is crucial during pregnancy, and you can always add water or coconut water to your smoothies for extra hydration.

These snacks and smoothies are a great way to ensure you're getting a steady intake of

essential nutrients. Keep them handy for when
you need a quick, healthy boost throughout the
day.

Conclusion

As you've turned the pages of *FamilyPro Guide to Pregnancy Nutrition and Diet*, you've gained more than just knowledge— you've empowered yourself to make confident, informed choices for your health and your baby's development. This book has equipped you with the tools to navigate every trimester with practical advice, science-backed meal plans, and real-world tips tailored to your needs. From understanding key nutrients to crafting balanced meals, you now have a roadmap to nourish your body and nurture your growing baby.

But a book is only as effective as its application. To truly maximize the benefits of what you've learned, remember to revisit the sections that resonate most with your needs at different stages of pregnancy. Save the recipes, build meal plans that work for your lifestyle, and lean on the strategies for managing cravings or addressing special dietary concerns. The goal is progress, not perfection—small, consistent efforts will make a big impact.

You're doing an incredible job, not just for yourself but for the new life you're creating. Trust your instincts, stay curious, and use this book as a foundation for making choices that feel right for you. Your dedication to a healthy pregnancy is an inspiring step toward a bright future for your baby.

If this book has helped you on your journey, please consider leaving a review. Your feedback not only supports this work but also helps other expectant mothers discover resources that can make a meaningful difference in their lives. Reviews are a powerful way to share your story and spread the word.

If you've enjoyed this book, be sure to check out other titles in the **FamilyPro series**. From postpartum nutrition to toddler meal planning, each book is designed to meet you where you are and guide you with practical, easy-to-follow advice.

As you step forward, remember: each choice you make is an act of love and care for yourself and your baby. Thank you for allowing this book to be part of your journey.